Teepa Snow's

When is Enough, Enough?

A Positive Approach to Finding Balance in a Caring Life

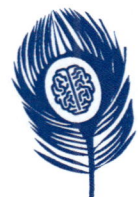

Teepa Snow • Christine Browdy • Dan Bulgarelli

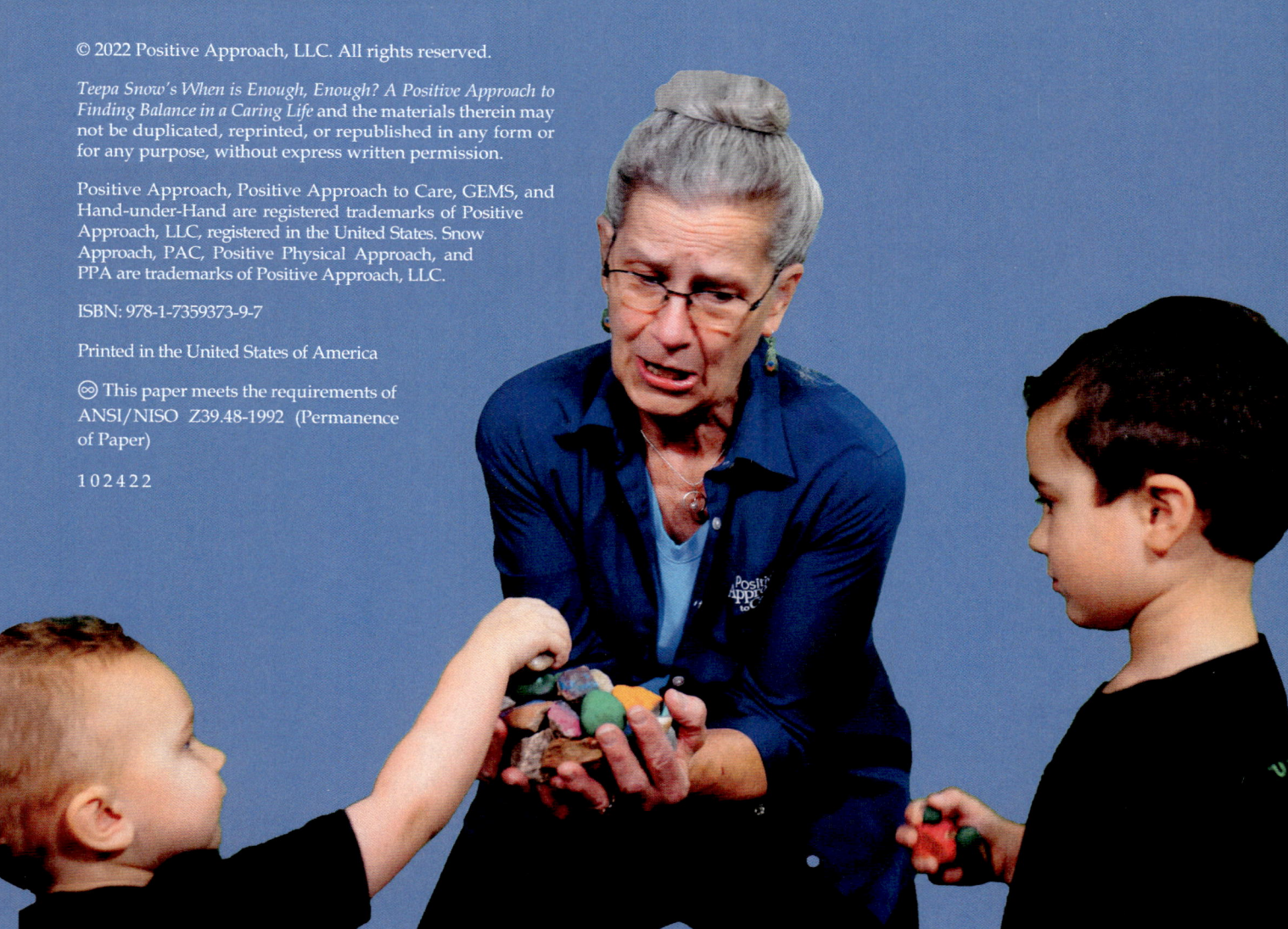

© 2022 Positive Approach, LLC. All rights reserved.

Teepa Snow's When is Enough, Enough? A Positive Approach to Finding Balance in a Caring Life and the materials therein may not be duplicated, reprinted, or republished in any form or for any purpose, without express written permission.

Positive Approach, Positive Approach to Care, GEMS, and Hand-under-Hand are registered trademarks of Positive Approach, LLC, registered in the United States. Snow Approach, PAC, Positive Physical Approach, and PPA are trademarks of Positive Approach, LLC.

ISBN: 978-1-7359373-9-7

Printed in the United States of America

∞ This paper meets the requirements of ANSI/NISO Z39.48-1992 (Permanence of Paper)

102422

Meet the Authors

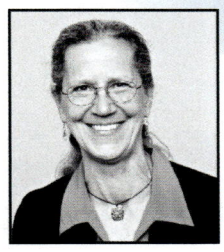

Teepa Snow: Our (My) goal with this guide is not to be right, but to be helpful. You will be the person who determines what is right for you, and when enough is enough… for you!

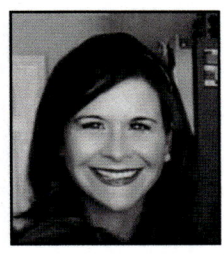

Christine Browdy: Deciding that you are ready to take the next step or figure something out requires courage and a willingness to look in the mirror. The journey of this guide has been one of growth, acceptance, and realizing that the needs we have matter and are important. My hope is that this guide will help you identify one thing that you might be willing to try, shift, or change.

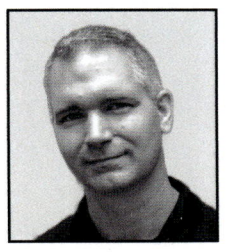

Dan Bulgarelli: I wrestled with the concept of enough for quite some time when the idea was brought to me. How do you define enough? It led me down a road of self-exploration, and at times, I felt exposed—but only to myself. Thankfully, I had Christine and Teepa to lean on, and I feel like I have a better understanding of enough and myself. I hope this book and the subsequent resources will be as helpful to you as they are to me.

Table of Contents

SECTION 1: Finding Balance — 07

SECTION 2: Being Balanced — 39

SECTION 3: Staying Balanced — 73

Introduction

Enough. Wow! A lot of different meanings all wrapped into one six letter word. Interesting that this one word can build someone up with purpose, value, and worth, and the same word, **when used differently**, can cause someone to crumble, feel lonely, invisible, and pushed aside. This word can be used with a tone of satisfaction and contentment, or frustration and disappointment.

Whatever came to your mind when you first saw the topic of this guidebook, **we get it**, we really do. Our goal with this book is to **help you examine enough** and all its many possible meanings and variations as we each journey through our lives. At times we do it alone, at times with others, with moments of pleasure and times of hardship.

You will see that, together, we will explore the concepts that surround humans and the idea of enough. Am I smart enough? Skilled enough? Aware enough? Kind enough?

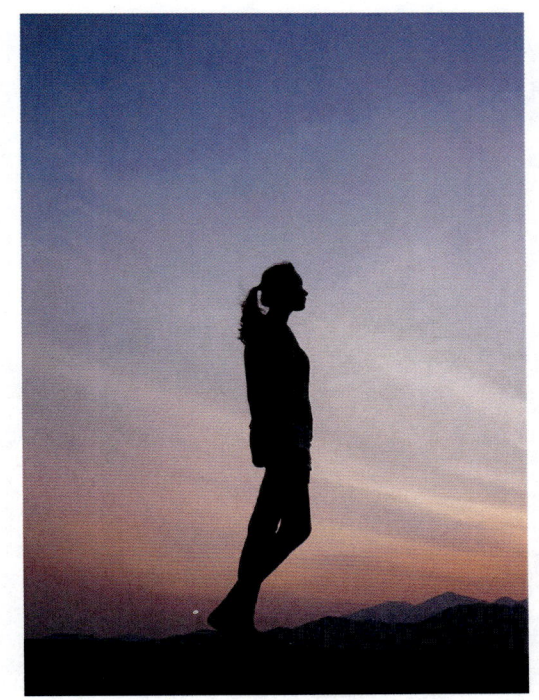

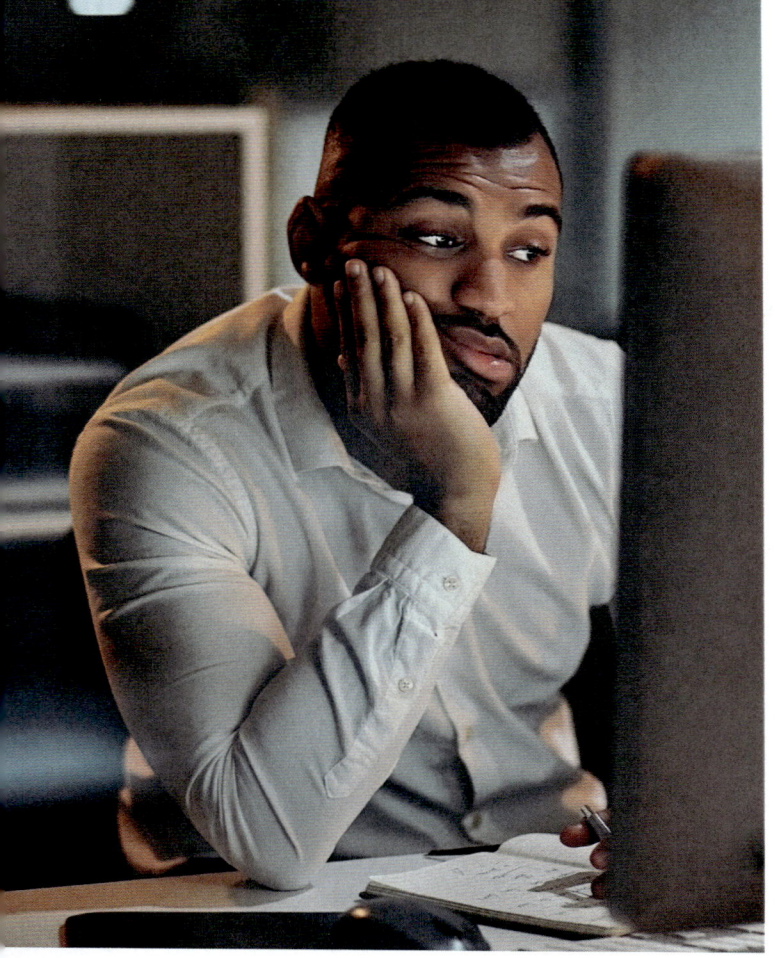

Doing enough? How would I know? Do I have more than enough? If so, how do I think or feel about that, and what can I do about it to get to **a just right** place? Let something go? Offer it or gift it to someone else? Store it away and carry it around with me, just in case? How might that work out?

Hopefully, these questions get your brain interested and curious, or maybe put your guard up. Either way, maybe we have said enough!

This guidebook is designed to offer new ways of seeing, thinking, feeling, and being when it comes to measuring enough, and finding balance. Maybe you would say that you are balanced, content, and satisfied with your life and what is around you. Or perhaps, you have had so many people in your life imply or tell you that you are not enough, it has become something that you believe about yourself.

Is the thought of uncovering some of that too much? That can be extremely uncomfortable, and to be honest, we have felt that way, too. We invite you to join us and trust this **journey for what it can be, and what is possible.**

Right now might be a good time for a deep breath. Take a minute and think about what we just talked about before going any further, and remember,

you do not have to do this alone. We are sure glad that we do not have to, either.

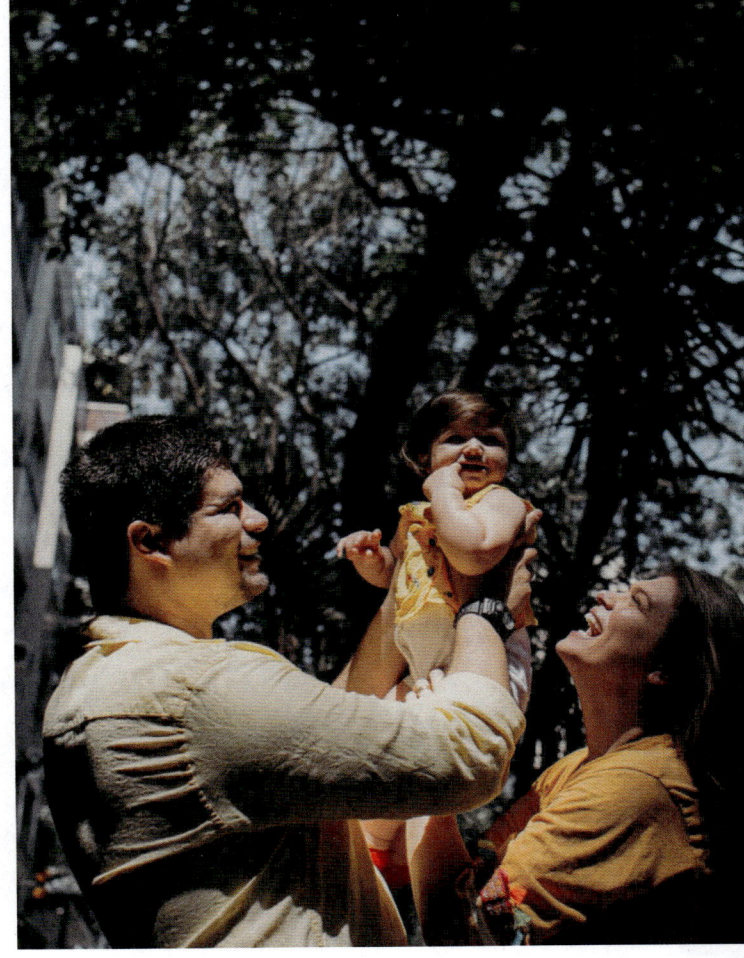

When is Enough, Enough? *A Positive Approach to Finding Balance in a Caring Life*

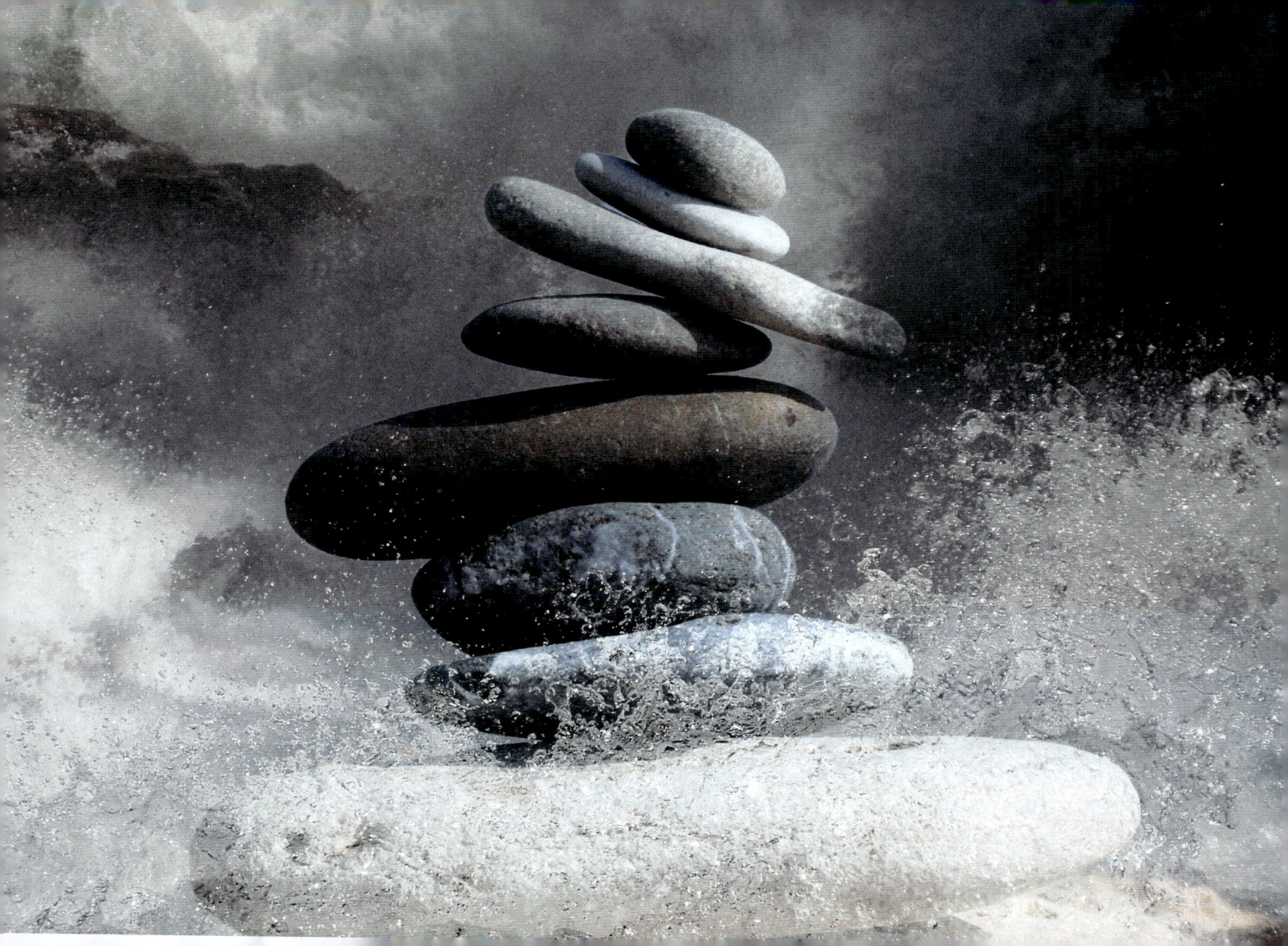

SECTION 1
Finding Balance

When you do not feel like you are doing enough, perhaps just thinking this means you are doing more and caring more than you realize.

What is Enough?

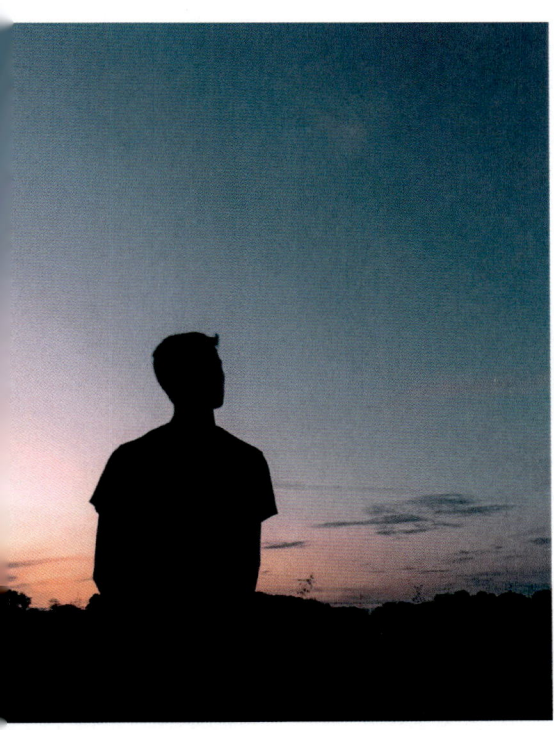

If things do not feel or seem right, then something is not balanced. So, how do we find balance, and how do we stay balanced? We can take an important step towards getting life in balance, after we are able to consider what we have enough of, what we have too much of, and what we do not have enough of.

So, what is enough? As you can probably tell by the subtitle and beginning of this book, we are looking at enough as being balanced. But what does enough mean? By definition, it means an acceptable amount, but that is just as vague, isn't it? When we look at things we like, we can have too little, enough, more than enough, or too much. For things we might not like as much, such as stress or pain, there really is not an amount that we would consider too little, or is there for you? Maybe there is none, an amount I can handle, and too much.

Finding a balance for anything can be difficult. We can often feel like we do not have enough of what we think we should have, or too much of what we do not want. Are these accurate feelings, or something else? How can we find out?

Enough is relative to each person and each situation. Most people are uncomfortable with not having enough, not being enough, not getting enough, or having someone tell you that you are not enough. That is a hard place to be, it can isolate us from others, make us want to hide, or maybe go seeking something or someone else. **Hiding or seeking** are two primitive reactions that may help us to get what we want or cause us to lose what we already have.

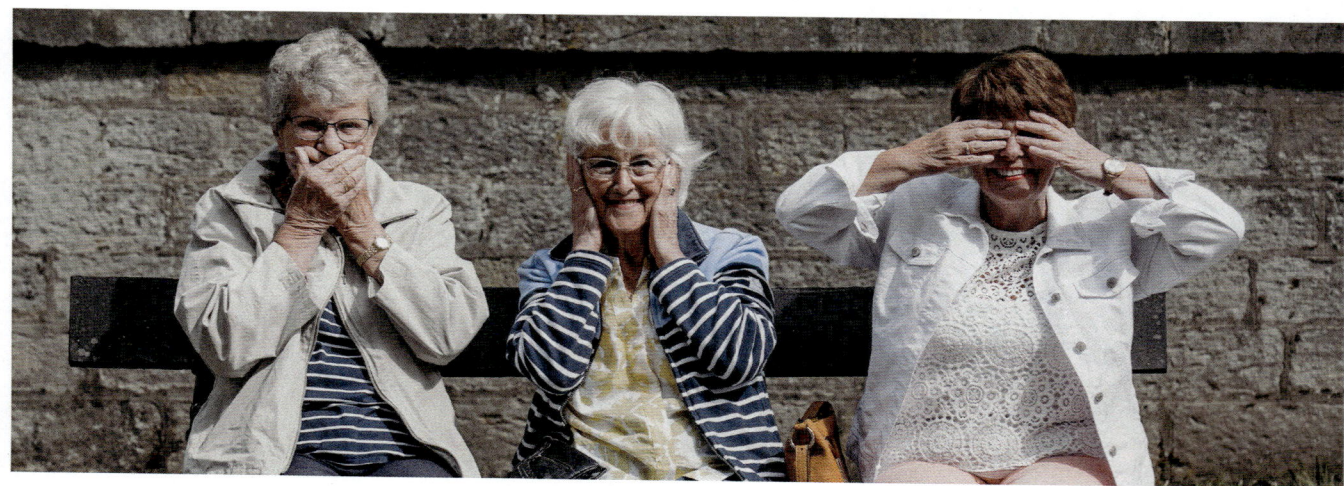

Needs. Likes. Wants.

As we continue our journey to finding enough, the just right amount or balance, it is **important to understand what we need.**

The word **need** is commonly misused. Here is an example. Do you really **need** a cup of coffee? Or do you **want** a cup of coffee because you are cold, tired, lonely, thirsty, or seeking a pause or break? Would a cup of coffee make you feel more comfortable in some way, or do you **like** the chemical rush you get from the caffeine in the coffee? Feel free to substitute the example of coffee with your favorite beverage.

Perhaps it is more of a question of **like or want** versus **need**.

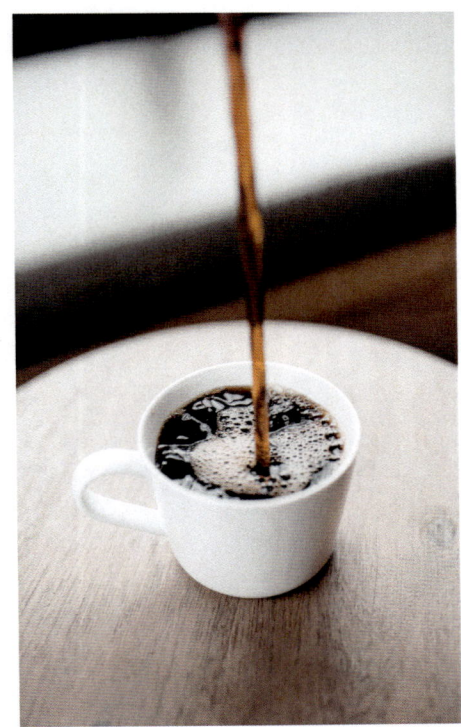

A little confusing? Try thinking of it this way. **Needs being met keep us alive**. **Likes and wants make life worth living.** Our body has certain needs that must be met in order to survive. The most primitive part of the brain is designed for survival by **seeking to get our needs met.** If our needs are not being met, we will do just about anything in order to fulfill what is necessary. However, if our basic needs are not in question, we can make choices based on our preferences, choosing things that bring us comfort and joy.

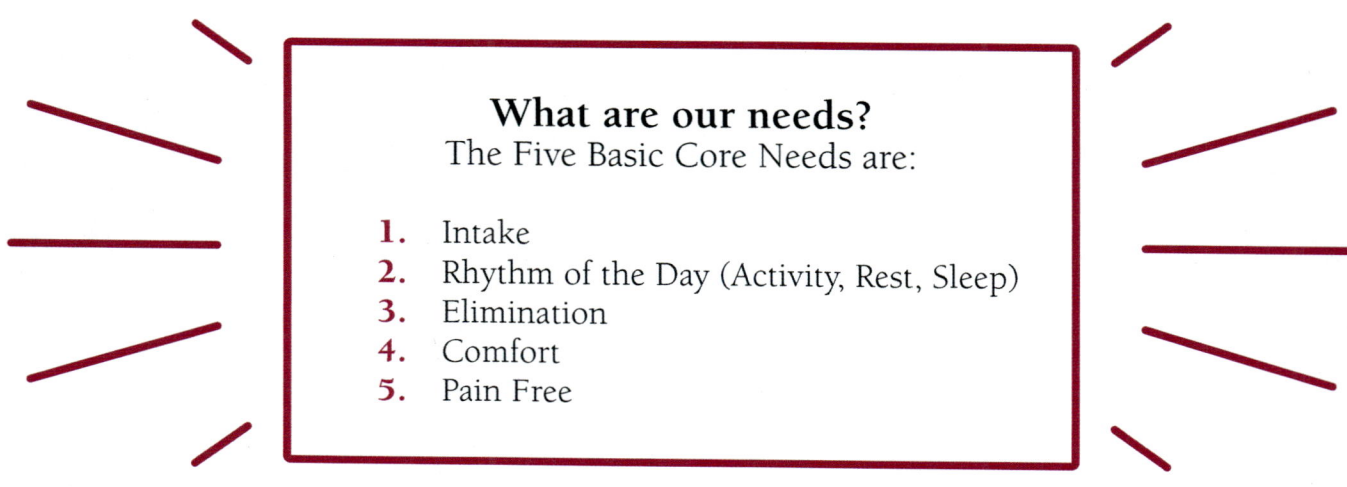

What are our needs?
The Five Basic Core Needs are:

1. Intake
2. Rhythm of the Day (Activity, Rest, Sleep)
3. Elimination
4. Comfort
5. Pain Free

We'll dive into this list in more detail in a few pages. However, to illustrate the differences between needs, likes, and wants, here is an example for the basic core need of intake.

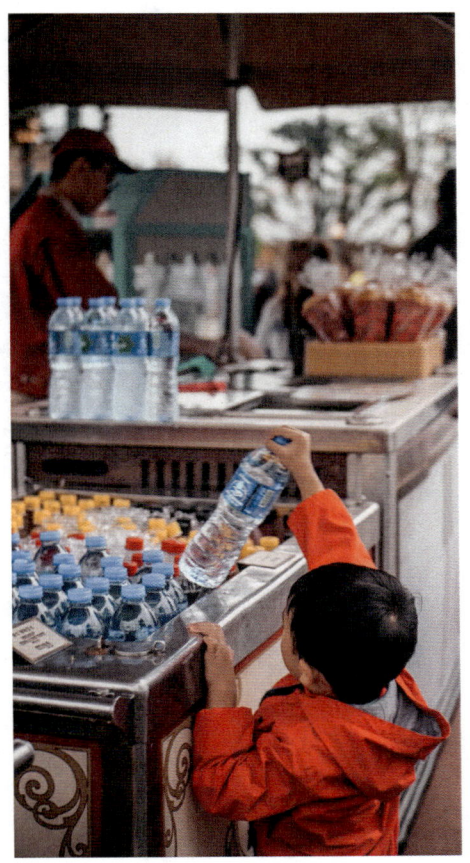

Intake – I need nourishment, food, and water, to survive. If I am in dire need and if my needs are not being met regularly, then it will not matter if the food tastes good or if the water is pure, my body is in need. For most of us, this need is met regularly, so we can choose the food we want and like because it tastes good or brings us comfort and joy. For hydration, I may choose bottled water, soda, or a sports drink instead of getting water from the tap because I prefer the taste. What are some examples of how you balance your needs with your likes and wants when it comes to food, drink, or even the aroma of the air?

The challenge is, for many people, **acquiring more of what we want and like**. How can we get comfortable with, and accept that there is a **medium point where we find balance, the just right amount?** On either end, we are working with too little or too much. This is where things can get tricky.

We don't want to merely **survive; we seek to thrive.** Ultimately, we want to do well and be able to develop and grow. However, **we can cease to thrive when we get too much of something, and it then becomes excess.** Humans are not meant to have excess; we are meant to have **just enough** so that we can thrive.

When is Enough, Enough? *A Positive Approach to Finding Balance in a Caring Life*

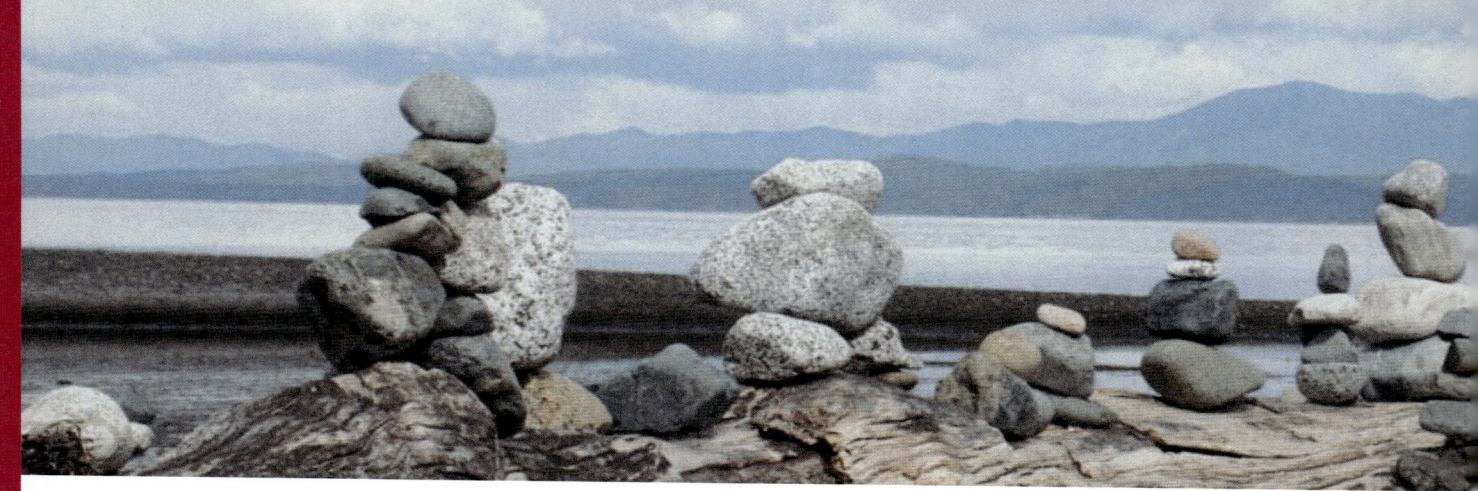

Have you ever found yourself gravitating to thinking in extremes? This is **too** hard, or this is **too** easy. But, what about this is **just right**? Have you ever acknowledged when something is just right?

With all of this, what we are doing is trying to get our needs, likes, and wants met, but sometimes all at the same time. Honestly, we tend to go overboard because it can be tough to acknowledge, and filter through, the differences between a need, a like, or a want.

When we have our needs met, and we are getting some of our likes and wants, **that means we are getting enough and can take what life throws at us.** We can recover from difficult situations, be flexible with the unexpected, and adapt to changes. **We are resilient because we can shift a little bit.**

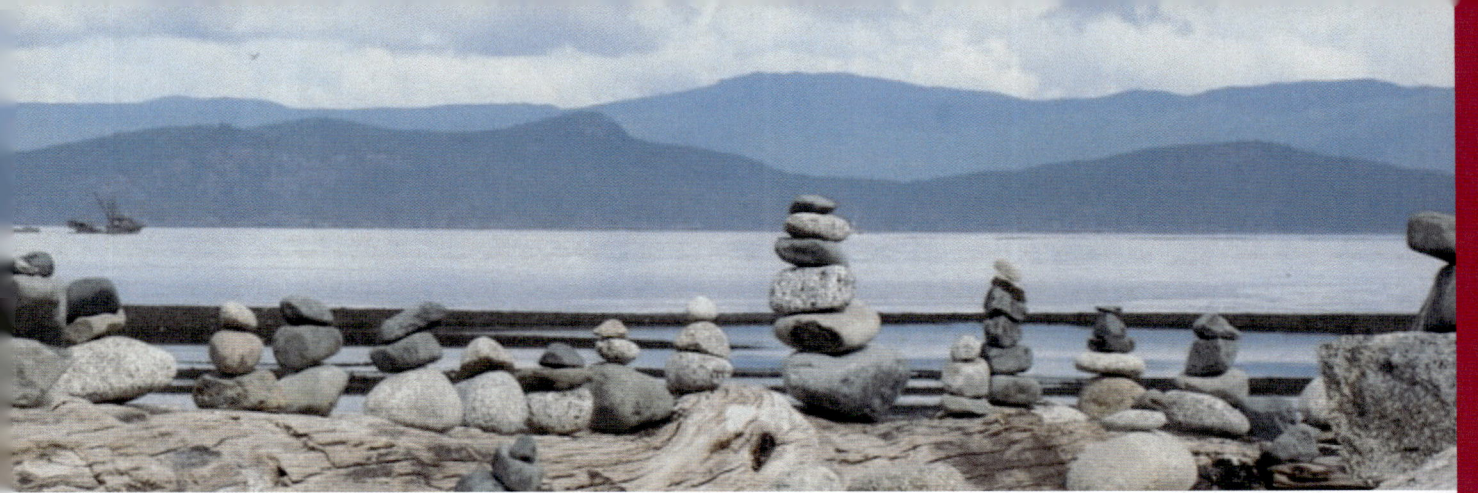

It is important to note, if we do not find a way to satisfy our basic core needs, and we do not participate in getting these basic needs met, we may endanger our very existence. **We will end up being unfulfilled and unbalanced with a feeling or thought of not having or being enough.** The tricky part is that by indulging in our likes and wants of the moment, our longer-term ability to thrive and even survive may take a major hit. An added variable when it comes to balance is the comparison of in this moment, and over a more extended period of time. **Hence the difference between a quick fix that doesn't last and a lifestyle change that is made for the duration.** So, if getting our basic needs met is the first step towards finding balance, how do we do that?

To live life every day we must at least feel like we have enough. If we do not, then we are in need. When a person is in need, relationships and life tend to get unbalanced.

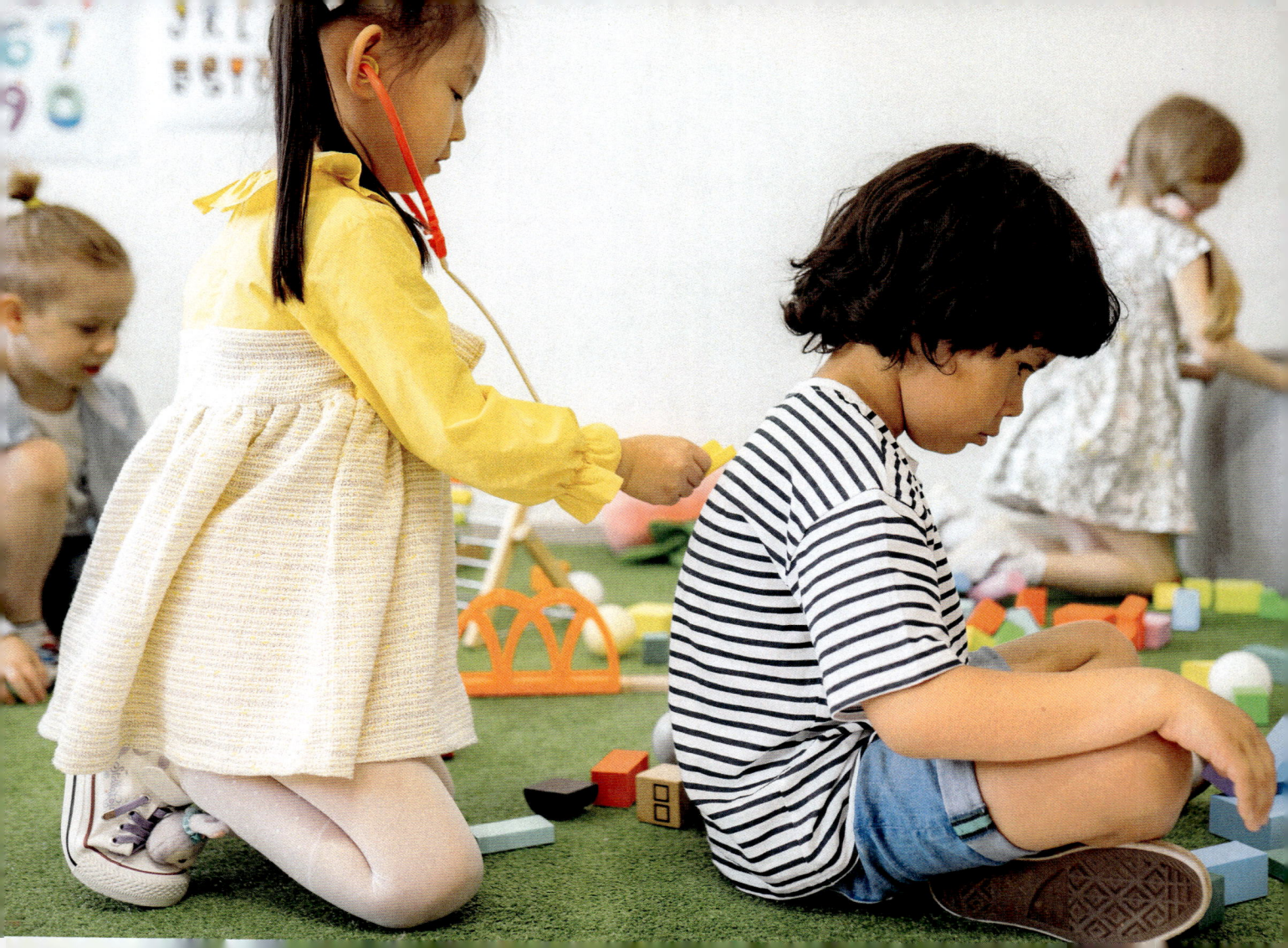

What is causing this need?

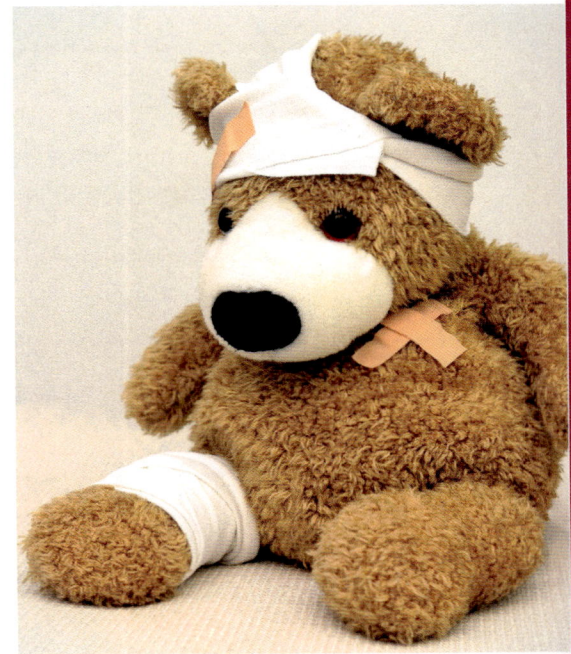

It is not always easy to determine where we have a need and what exactly is causing that need. It seems to be a little easier when the pain is physical, we can see it, touch it, and can often watch the process of healing. We observe or notice a change as a bruise, scratch, or broken bone gets better or worse. However, an emotional, mental, or spiritual wound seems harder to recognize or diagnose, much less accept and address.

Sometimes when we think we have a physical need, it might actually be something different. Something not as tangible, but certainly something as real. **A mental, emotional, or spiritual need, when not addressed can cause a physical problem, but the root of it remains mental, emotional, or spiritual.** If we only treat or address the symptom, we do not truly heal what caused it, which means it will eventually come back and can cause more trouble.

When is Enough, Enough? *A Positive Approach to Finding Balance in a Caring Life*

Depending on our past experiences, current situations, and personal beliefs, it is natural that we have different definitions of what is meant by physical, mental, emotional, and spiritual.

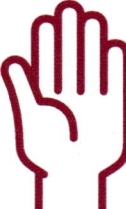

Physical – Our bodies. The health or condition of our bodies. Strength, movement, breath, vision, our senses, internal organs, brain, heart, liver, or anything above and under our skin, hair, nails, or teeth.

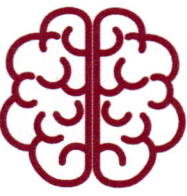

Mental – Our thought system. The ability to be creative, logical, or intellectual. To learn, be challenged, to think, process, strategically plan, move through a sequence, make a decision, understand consequences, or to consider a different perspective or point of view.

For the context of this guide, and from the perspective of uncovering our basic core needs, we invite you to consider these definitions and distinctions. Feel free to add your own spin to these if something does not fit for you.

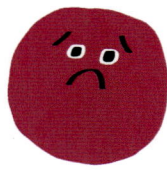

Emotional – Our feeling system. The ability to feel, express, and show happiness, sadness, love, hate, optimism, self-esteem, self-acceptance, loneliness, isolation, interest, disinterest, inclusion, or exclusion.

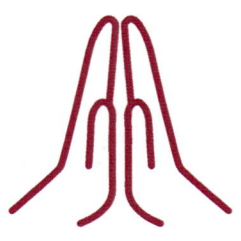

Spiritual – An internal set of beliefs, principles, and values that provide reason and guidance for one's life. It can be based on religious beliefs or on other beliefs and principles. It combines thought and emotion to form a base upon which to act or do things. It allows us the ability to seek and draw purpose and meaning from our lives, and can provide a sense of comfort, fulfillment, acceptance, value, peace, and security. It helps us connect with people and the world around us.

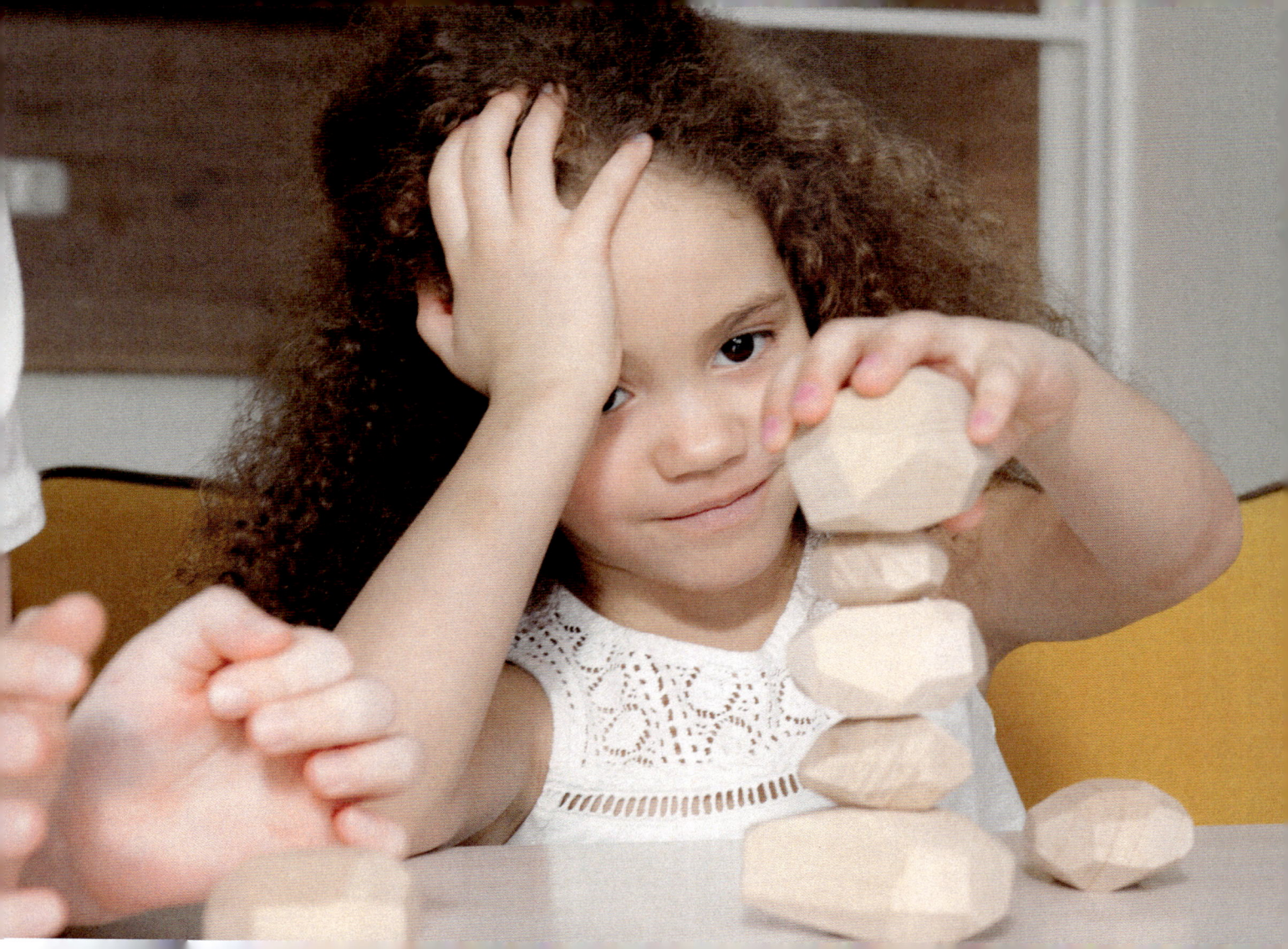

Remember, as we mentioned before, **when life seems out of balance or something is just not right, the root cause of it is usually an unmet need.** By breaking this down, we are laying a foundation for us to be able to find the source of the issue, rather than simply putting a temporary bandage over the symptom.

Let us now look deeper at each human need and identify some examples of how to meet each need.

As we mentioned previously, the **Five Basic Core Needs** are:

1. Intake
2. Rhythm of the day (Activity, Rest, Sleep)
3. Elimination
4. Comfort
5. Pain Free

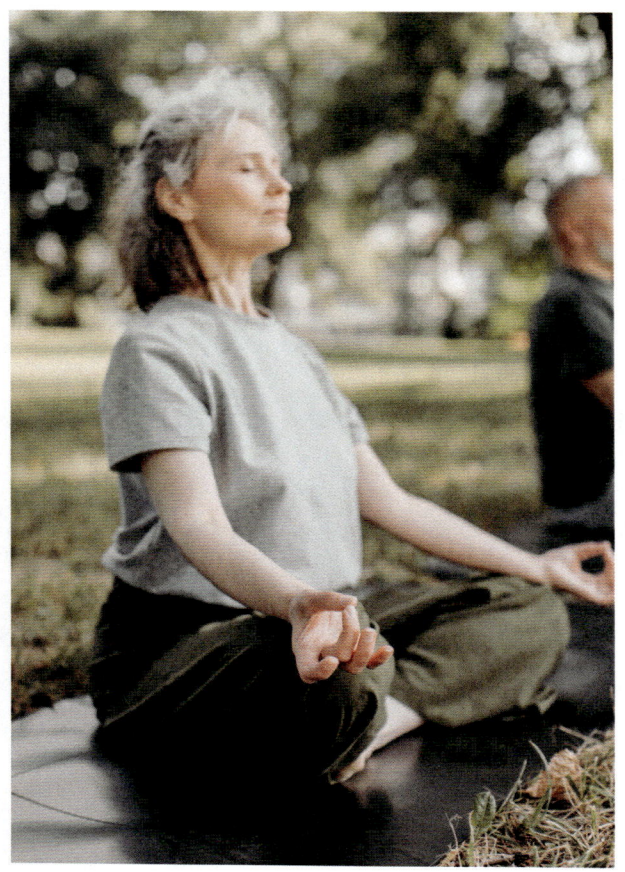

1
Intake –

To survive, humans must take enough in to be sustained and to live. **What we put in will eventually, in one way or another, come out.** So, what we allow into our bodies and lives might be worth looking into. We can take things in by:

Physical – Taking in oxygen, hydration, nourishment, medication, visual data, auditory data, sensory-motor data, smell, or taste data.

 Mental – Developing or participating in new information, new experiences, conversations that challenge us, thoughts, ideas, or memories of the past. Being creative.

 Emotional – Doing things we enjoy, activities or work that gives us purpose, meaning, value, or joy.

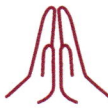 ***Spiritual*** – Gathering or participating in meditation, yoga, reading, prayer, positivity, connection, light, conversations and/or being with people who share our belief system, music, nature, or water. Receiving or accepting forgiveness.

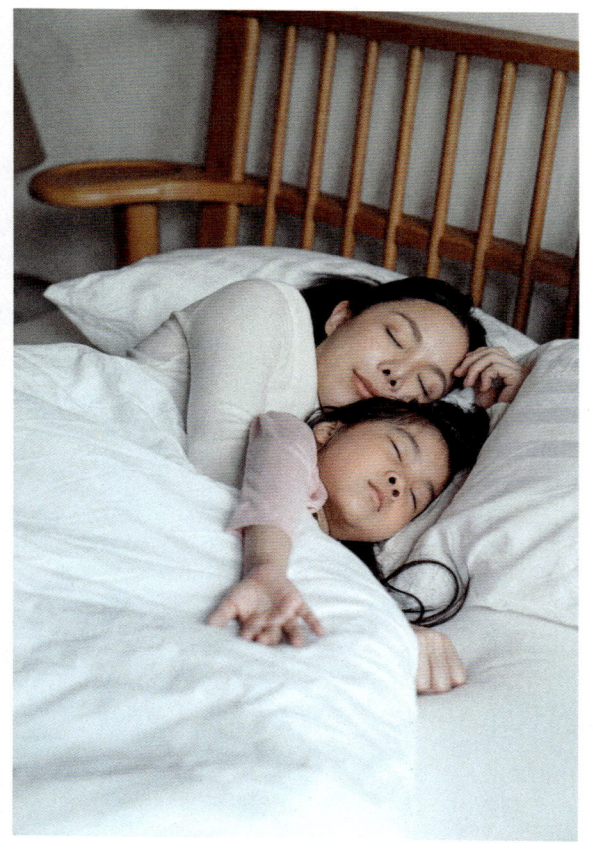

2

Rhythm of the Day (Activity, Rest, or Sleep) –

Taking care of the inside. Our bodies are designed and created with rhythm. This is related to circadian patterns. Our heartbeat, our breath, our daily patterns, our lives are all rhythmic. There are highs and lows, starts and stops, awake and asleep. **To be balanced, we must have times of the day when we are active, times of the day when we rest, and times when we sleep.** We are all different in how we do this. We can be active, at rest, or sleep by:

Physical – Making time for sleeping, resting, walking, or moving.

 Mental – Being intentional about thinking, working, or tuning out and taking a break.

 Emotional – Identify what causes you to feel burned out, exhausted, drained, stressed, or anxious.

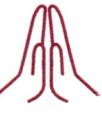 **Spiritual –** Thinking about what gives us a sense of meaningfulness and fulfillment in life and how to intentionally make time and space for that. Connecting with other people or participating in an activity based on the same belief system or reflecting peacefully, quietly.

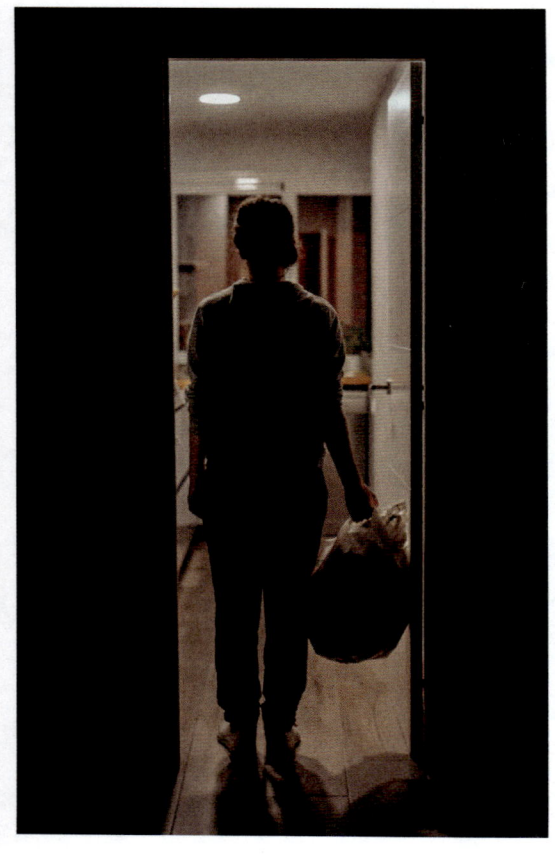

3

Elimination –

We must get rid of stuff we do not need, otherwise it just piles up around us or in us. We are not meant to keep and hold onto everything. **Letting go of something is not giving up.** This can be a very vulnerable position that we put ourselves in, which is why we can easily ignore this specific need. **Getting something out that we are holding in can have less negative power over us out in the open and in the light.** This is not always easy, but often creates quite a relief. We can eliminate things by:

 **Physical** – Releasing urine, carbon dioxide, tears, sweat, or feces. This can also be eliminating clutter in our environment or items around us that are not being used or just taking up space.

 Mental – Expressing painful, challenging thoughts, or sharing positive thoughts or encouragement with someone. Journaling, storytelling, writing a letter to someone that we give to them or destroy after it is written.

 Emotional – Is there a relationship that has become toxic? Perhaps someone has become a bad influence or has started to pull you away from what you know is right. Telling someone something that we have been holding on to or connecting in a new, different, or more honest way.

 **Spiritual** – Identifying and letting go of guilt, shame, or forgiving someone else or ourselves, which is not saying that what happened or was said was ok. It allows us to not have to carry the heavy burden of holding a grudge or the feeling of bitterness any longer. Music, conversation, or meditation. Getting away from noise and distraction or stepping out of aloneness and connecting with someone or something.

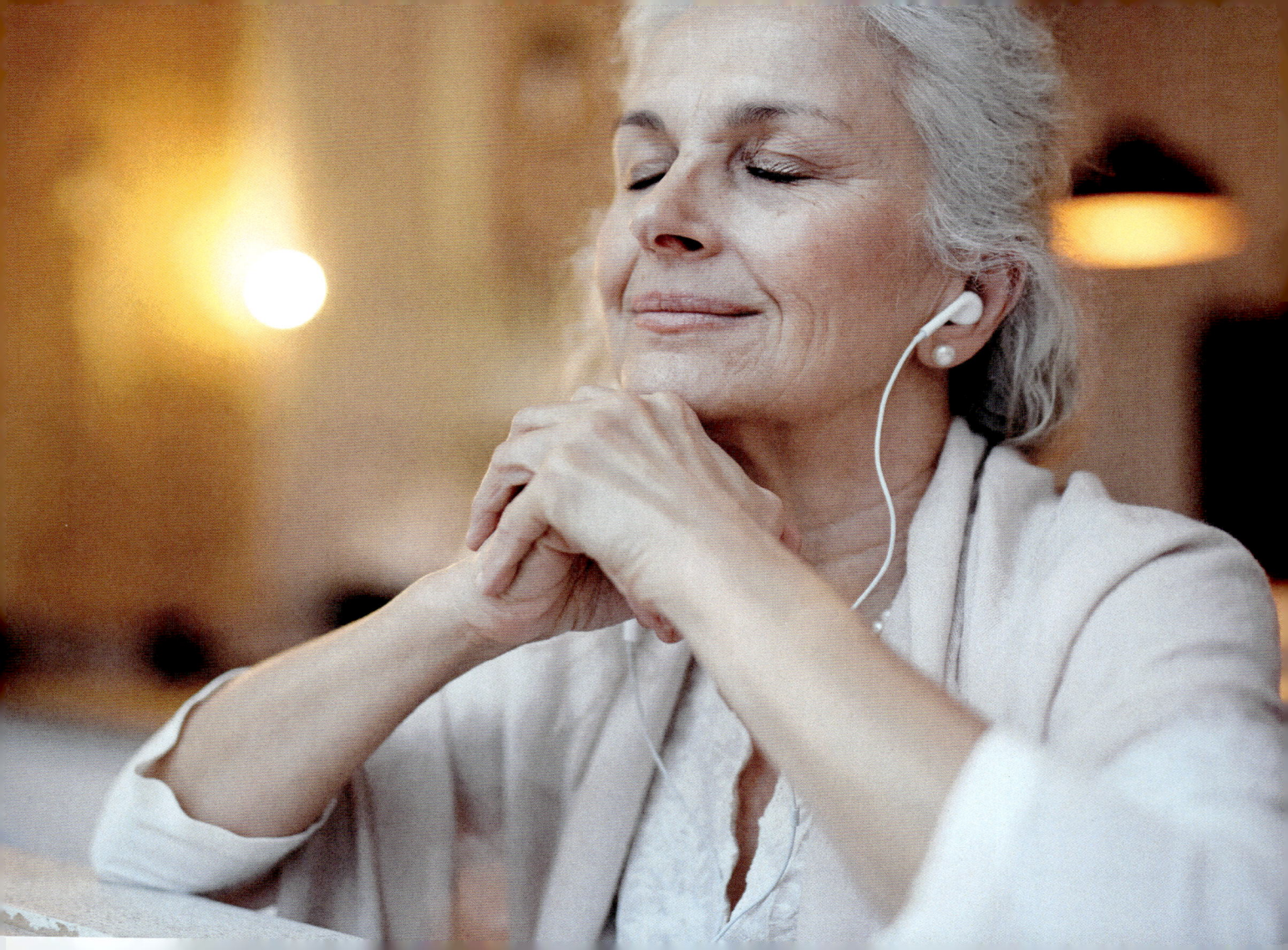

Let's pause here.

So far, we have talked about intake, rhythm of the day, and elimination. These are often easy to notice when the need is physical, but do we always notice when there is a mental, emotional, or spiritual need? We must allow ourselves to look hard at these first, before we can be prepared or ready to consider discomfort and pain. Discomfort and pain are strong, powerful, and can be tough to wrap our heads around. **But spending time looking into our needs of intake, rhythm of the day, and elimination can help us get to the root cause of our discomfort or pain.**

While reading this section, was the first person you thought of you, or someone else? Did someone else's unmet needs jump out at you? Well, they certainly might seem obvious on the surface, but as we are discovering, there is always more to the story. Let us look in the mirror first. We are talking about ways **we can meet our own unmet needs.** This is about us and what **we have the power and control to change.**

4

Comfort –

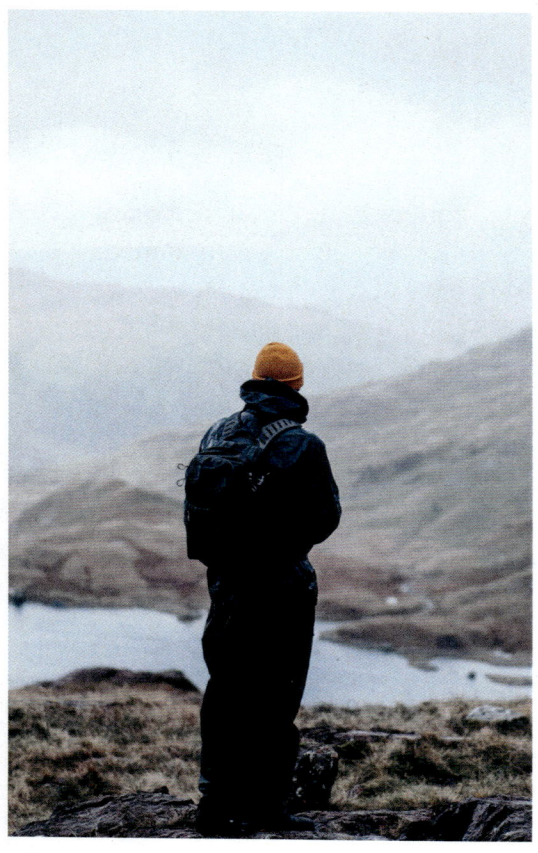

We must have a certain level of comfort with, and in ourselves, or we are **spending a lot of energy trying to find peace and get comfortable.** How do we get enough comfort so that we are content, but not so much that we are too comfortable and do not want to do anything? For some, being too comfortable can hinder our desire to do anything. Being uncomfortable, on the other hand, can lead us into the action of hiding or seeking. We might hide from what is making us uncomfortable without addressing it or seek something new and different. We can get the right amount of comfort by:

 ***Physical –*** Choosing clothing or environment that is pleasing to our senses. Clothing that is a preferred texture and temperature, soft, coarse, warm, or cool. Sitting in a chair that is firm, swivels, or rocks, or one that is cushioned. Adjusting the room temperature so that is not too cool, not too warm, but just right.

 Mental – Taking a pause during a stressful moment or conversation. Stepping back, taking a slow deep breath in, and slowly letting it out. Consider who you are with and if you can be yourself around them, or is it someone who expects you to be a different way? Practicing a conversation or an interaction with someone before it occurs or including an additional support person to be involved.

 Emotional – Choosing to find a positive perspective or outlook. Identifying something to be grateful for. Consider acknowledging the value of having an authority figure, expert, or mentor involved to help process a difficult interaction or situation.

 ***Spiritual –*** Reflecting on or seeking how we feel or how we think we are connected to the world, people, and nature around us. Consider exploring what creates meaning, value, purpose, and worth. Perhaps doing this in a community/partnership, or alone depending on what makes us most comfortable.

Scan this code with your smartphone's camera
or visit **www.teepasnow.com/resources/enough-guide**
on your computer.

When is Enough, Enough? *A Positive Approach to Finding Balance in a Caring Life*

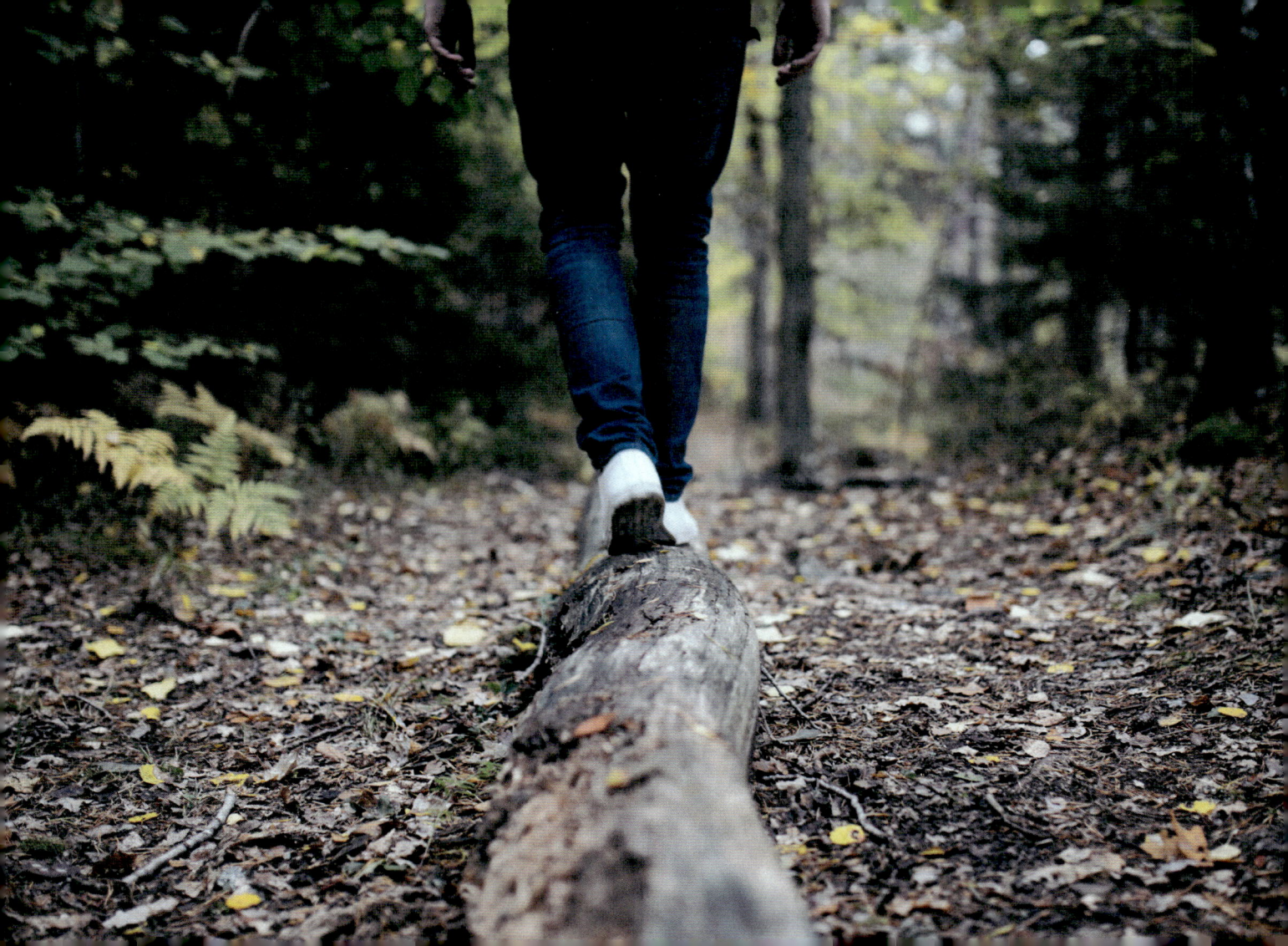

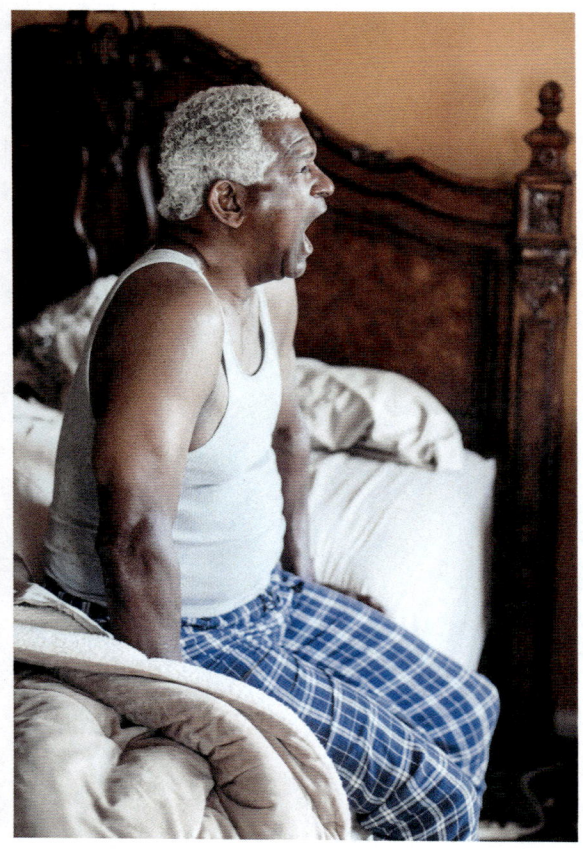

5

Pain Free –

Many times we experience pain before we realize that we have an unmet need. When we let discomfort go too far, it begins to hurt. That hurt or pain can be physical, mental, emotional, or spiritual. **Humans naturally seek to avoid pain, but there is often a level of discomfort we can accept if it seems worth it.** If discomfort goes to such an extent that it becomes pain, we may start to avoid it or get to a point of having to get rid of it. We might throw everything away because it hurts too much. We can seek to be pain free by:

 ***Physical*** – Listening to our bodies and having an awareness of subtle or sudden changes. Seeking support and medical attention when something is not right or becomes uncomfortable. Choosing ways to maintain regular checkups or health monitoring.

 Mental – Intentionally taking a break from what is stressful, even a moment or two can be helpful. Acknowledging that the situation we are in is difficult, or hard.

 Emotional – Being willing to acknowledge and be honest about what we are feeling. This may mean being vulnerable, which is a very courageous thing to do. At times, it may mean letting go of relationships or interactions that are causing pain or finding the right support that will keep the discomfort from shifting into pain.

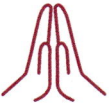 ***Spiritual*** – Identifying what we think about spirituality or the meaning of human existence. Being honest and open about what draws us to connecting with life or what has caused us to not want to be, feel, or think we are connected.

Are you in pain or are you uncomfortable? Consider giving some thought to this, because sorting it out is very important. When something really hurts, putting a bandage on it or trying to kiss it to make it better it is not going to be enough.

Looking at the source versus focusing on the symptoms is a critical step when choosing to move forward.

Figuring out what is causing the pain, and where the pain is coming from is the only way to begin to heal. Until we can identify the pain, describe the pain, unpack the pain, figure out how deep it goes, and where it is coming from, it is going to be hard to get anything else to help.

Whew! We uncovered a lot of things in this section. Some of it might be easy to consider, while some of it might be very challenging. It is important to remember that we, as humans, have basic needs that must be met. **When we do not get our needs met, we become unbalanced and can become distressed.**

Remember, **needs being met keep us alive, while likes and wants make life worth living.** We will always have needs, but how do we balance having likes and wants without going to a place that is too much for too long? On the other hand, how can we think about our tolerances for things like discomfort, pain, sadness, anger, or stress? These are all, inevitably, part of life.

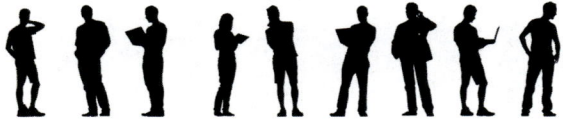

The answer to all these questions will be different for each person, of course. When was the last time you looked at yourself in relation to these aspects to think about them rationally? Only when you look at **your needs** can you honestly say that something is a need versus a want or a like. Just because something is a like or a want does not mean it is inherently bad, but recognizing it is the first step to balancing it.

Look at what you see as the negatives in your life and how do you find a balance between what you can handle and still recover and thrive versus what is **Just. Too. Much.**

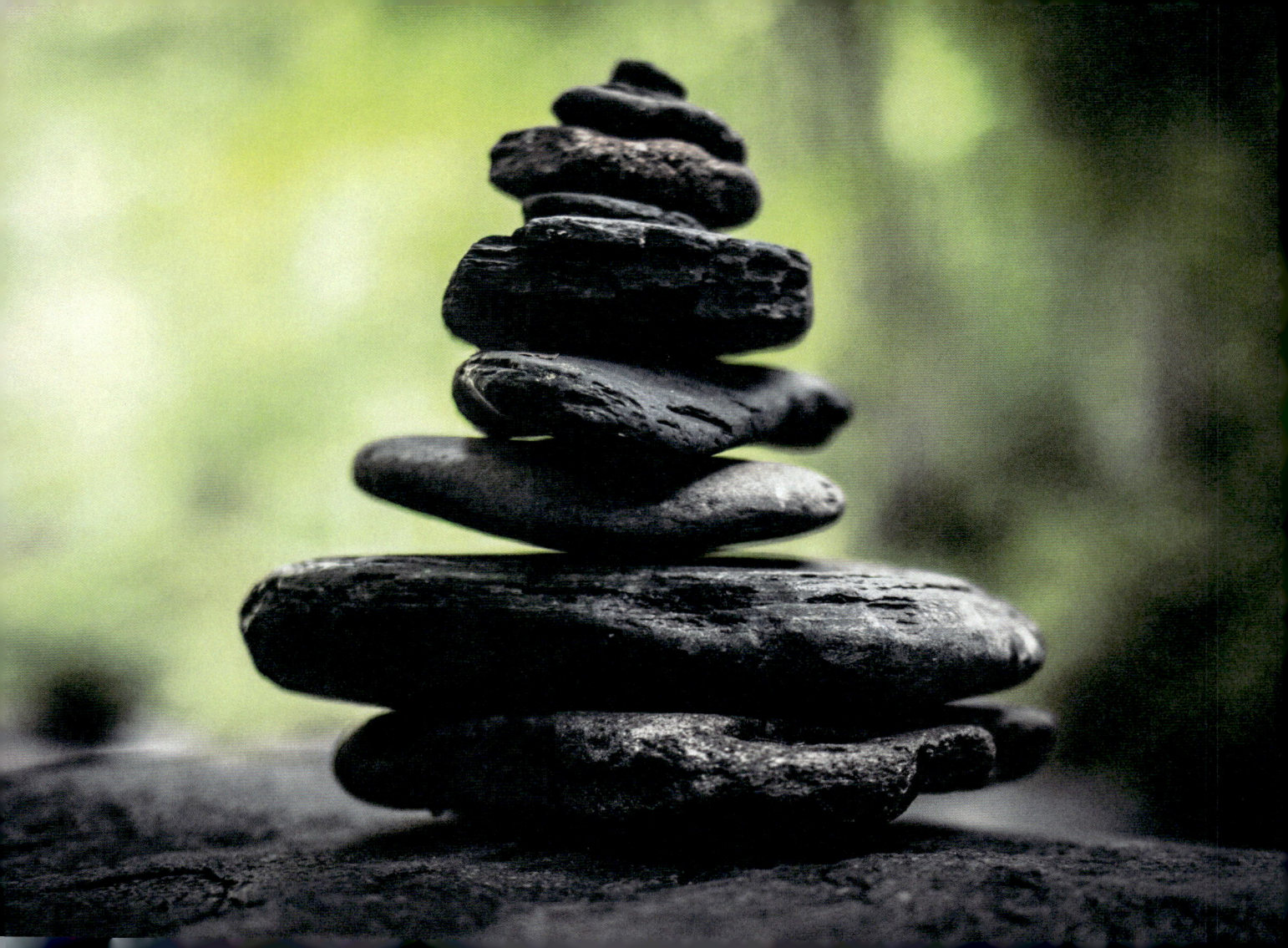

SECTION 2
Being Balanced

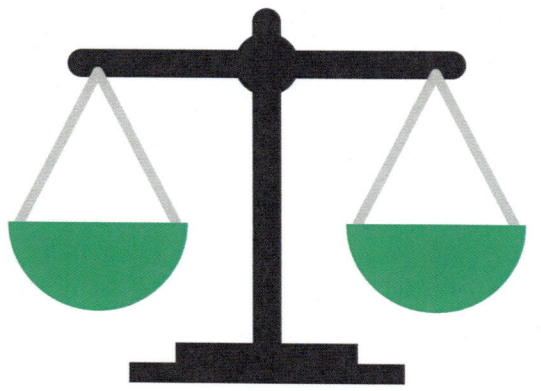

In all things, there must be a balance.

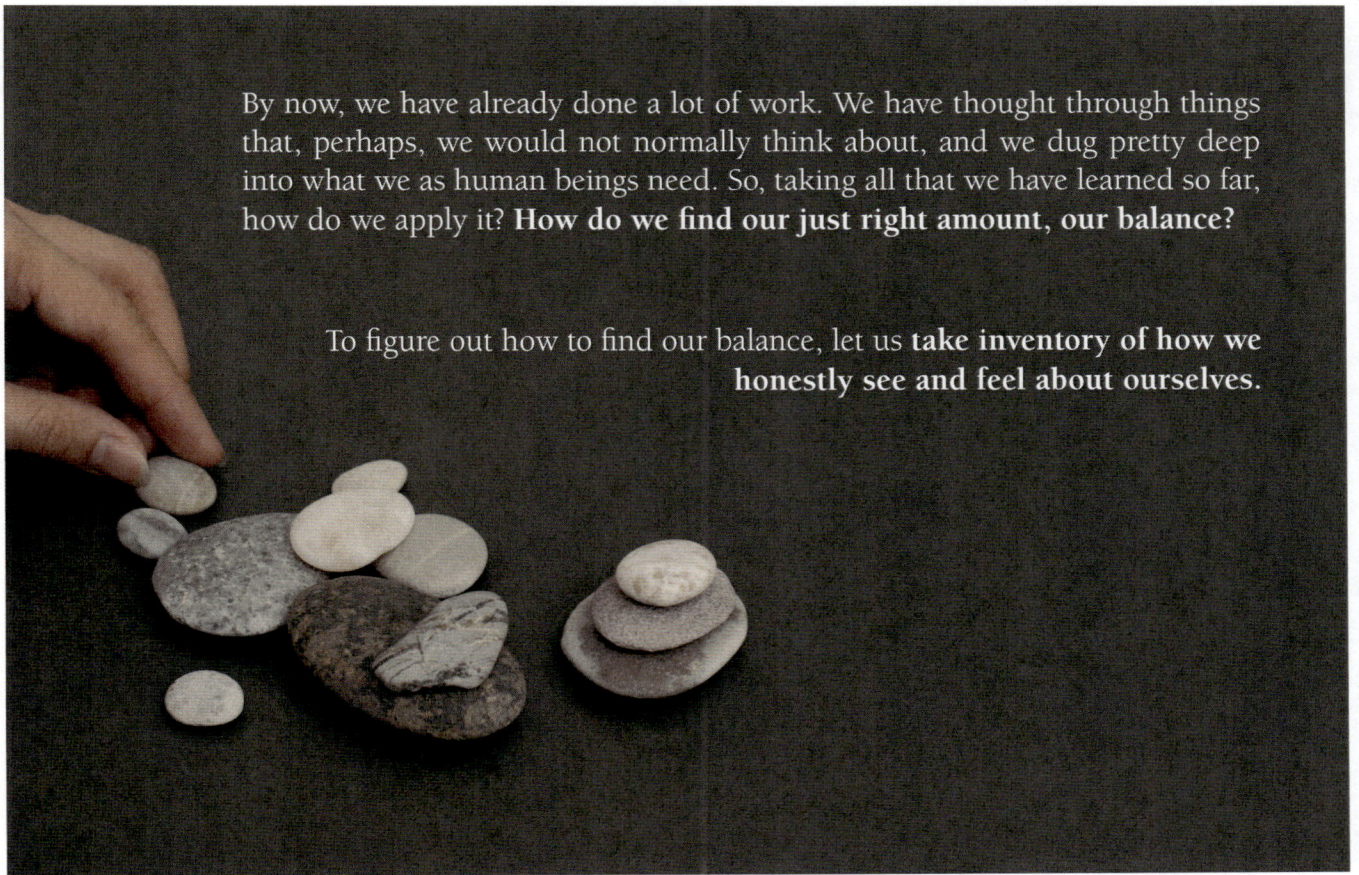

By now, we have already done a lot of work. We have thought through things that, perhaps, we would not normally think about, and we dug pretty deep into what we as human beings need. So, taking all that we have learned so far, how do we apply it? **How do we find our just right amount, our balance?**

To figure out how to find our balance, let us **take inventory of how we honestly see and feel about ourselves.**

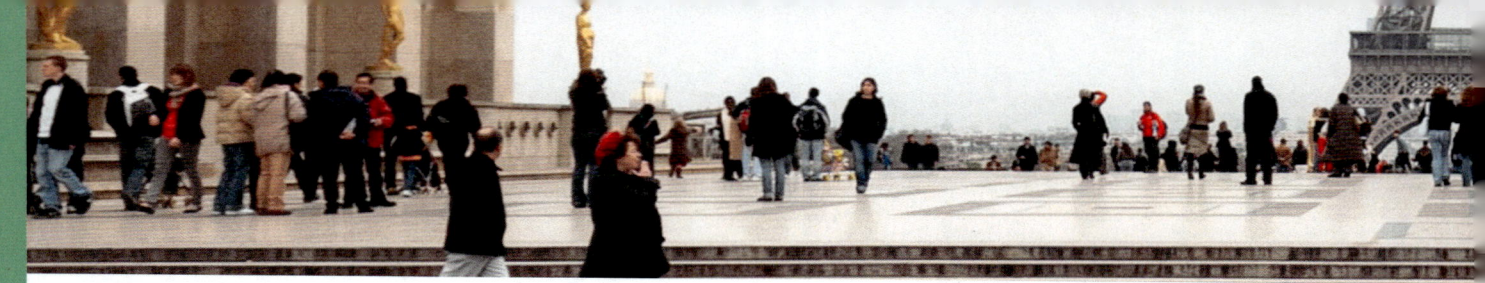

How often do you pause and think about yourself? Hmm, interesting question. At times you may be intensely focused on some aspect of yourself, and yet miss the bigger picture of how you are doing overall. **A few examples might be:**

- Meeting your weight goal, focusing only on the number on the scale, but losing sight of your overall health.

- Buying the perfect pair of running shoes, piece of exercise equipment, or yard tool and not making or taking the time to use them consistently.

- Knowing you need more sleep, so you get into bed earlier, but spend time scrolling on your phone, watching another episode of a show, or reading another chapter of a book before actually going to sleep.

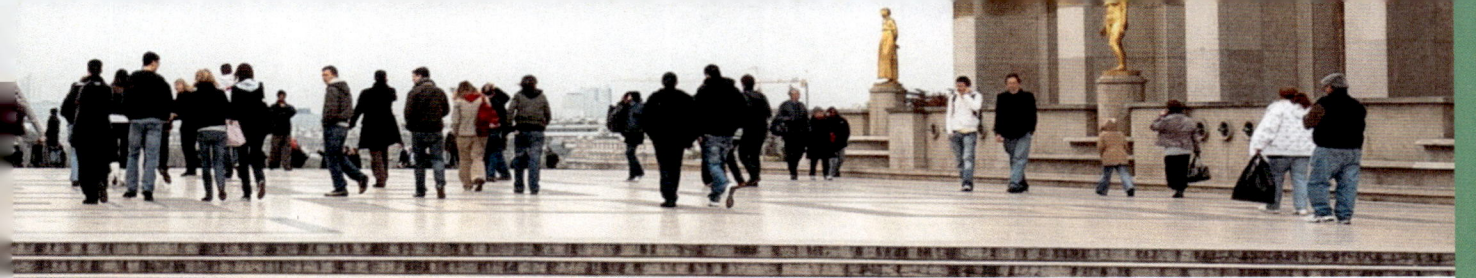

If it seems that it has been a while since you have thought about yourself, could it be because of one of these reasons?

- Maybe you are caring for someone living with dementia. Maybe you are caring for children. Maybe you have a role in your job that requires a lot of your time and attention.

- Maybe you have always put other people before yourself.

- Maybe the thought of spending time on yourself causes a feeling of guilt.

- Maybe it seems like there just is not enough time to think about yourself because there are so many demands placed on you.

- Maybe the exhaustion is just too great, the hurt too deep, or the fear too gripping.

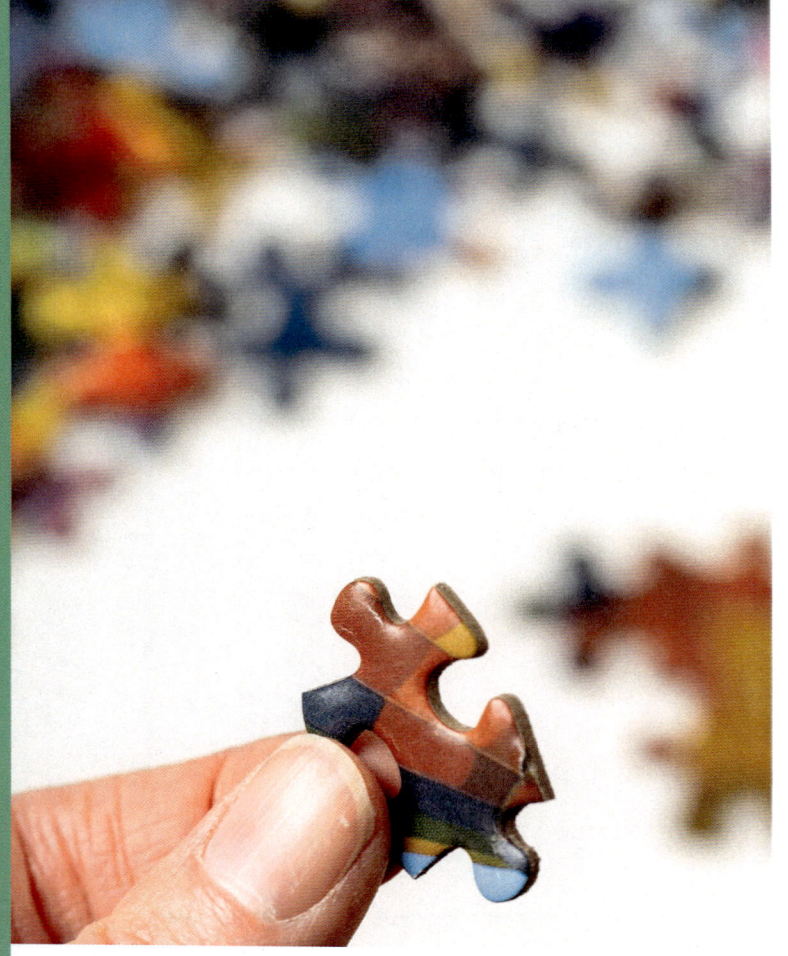

If any of this sounds familiar, you are not alone. Sometimes, we need permission to look in the mirror and

ask ourselves if we are getting what we need, are we enough, do we have enough, or are we getting too much of something.

Sometimes it is helpful to take a step back, look at the big picture and not focus too much on pieces of our life, but consider how we are doing overall.

Source of the Message

A very important part of looking in the mirror and figuring out if we are or have enough, is considering the source of the message that we are choosing to believe.

External – Someone else said or is saying that we are not enough or do not have enough, or societal expectations that might be placed on us. Generated from without.

Internal – Our internal awareness and beliefs about ourselves that drive us. Self-generated or created from within.

Mixed – A combination of external and internal. Our interpretation of what other people may or may not think of us. For some, an internal belief is directly related to external feedback, options, or assessments, regardless of whether it is true.

What do you believe to be true about yourself? Take a few moments to write your thoughts or feelings down here. Consider the five categories of human needs when you complete this process so as not to limit your self-regard.

_____

_____

_____

_____

_____

_____

_____

_____

Now, ask yourself where those words came from or are coming from. Did someone tell you something, say something to you, or about you that formed the way you see yourself? Is it society's expectations of you that can feel overwhelming or confirm your thoughts? Is it something else entirely?

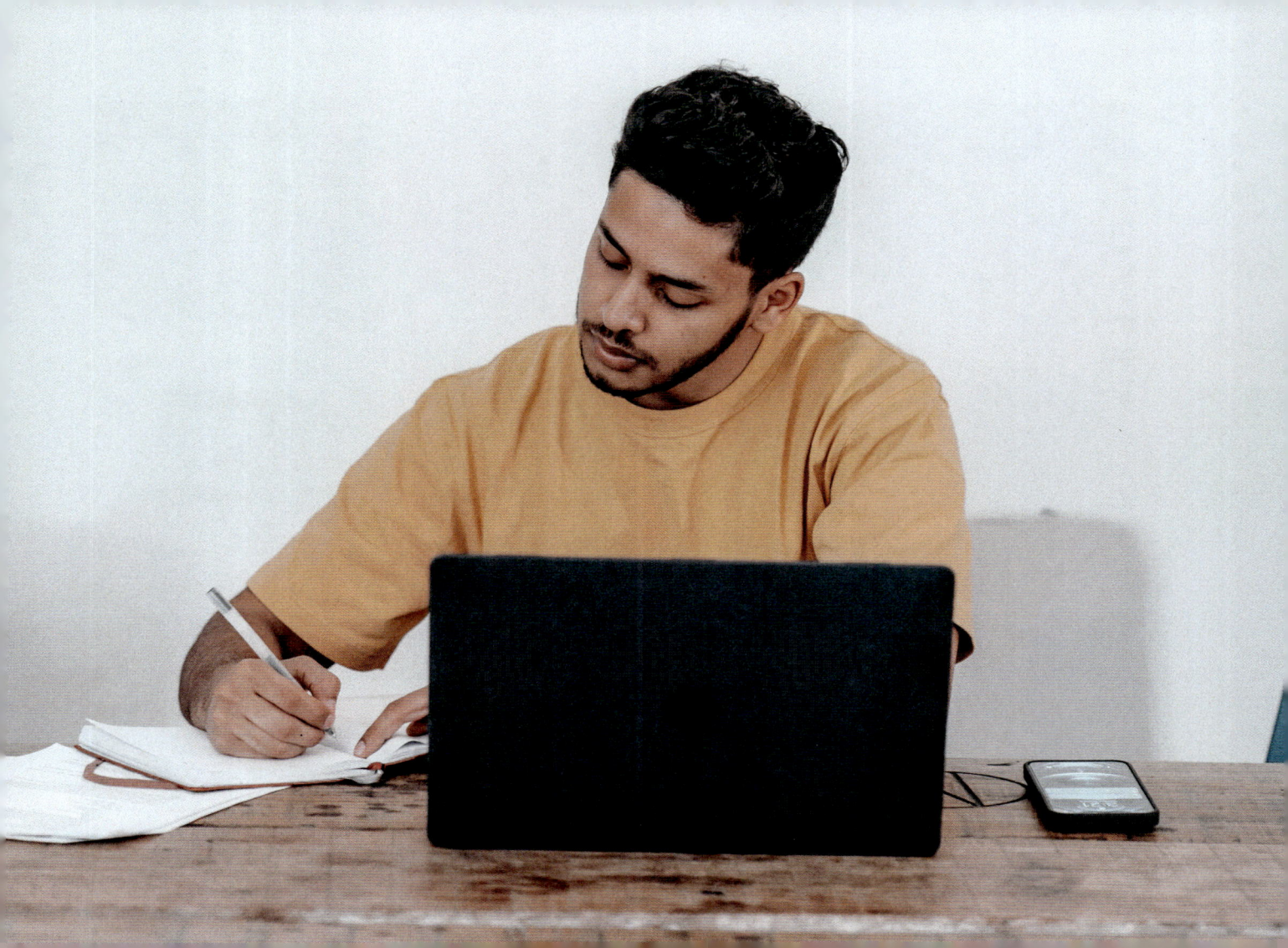

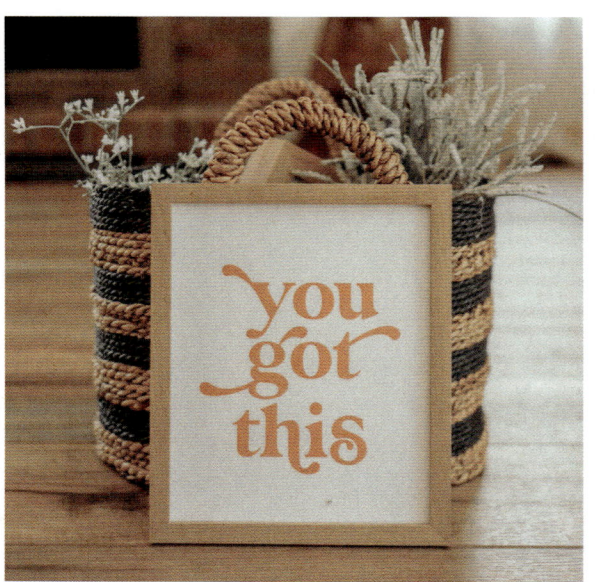 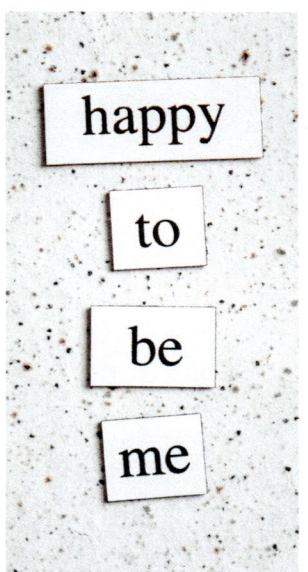 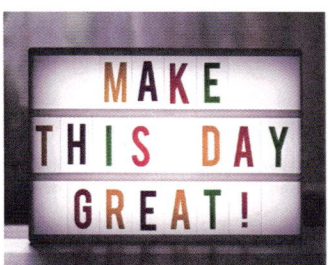 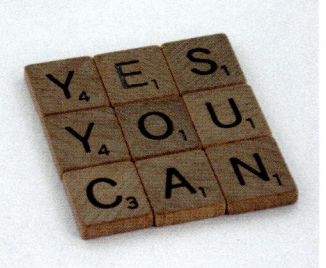

Words spoken to us or about us have the power to either build us up and fill us with life or tear us down and crumble us. So often, as adults, **we grow into what someone once said we would or should become.** We often hold onto what we hear spoken to or about us. If you remember words spoken to you filling you with comfort, joy, affirmation, fulfillment, and self-worth, **be thankful for the type of positivity** that you were taking in or currently are taking in.

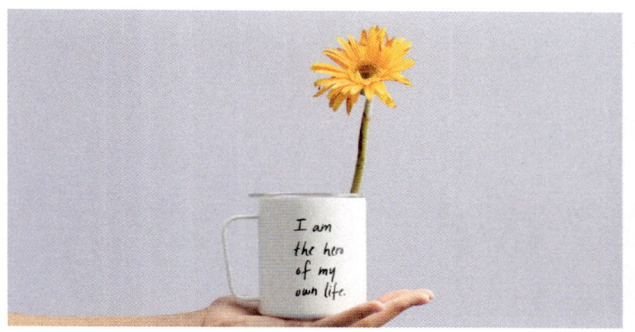 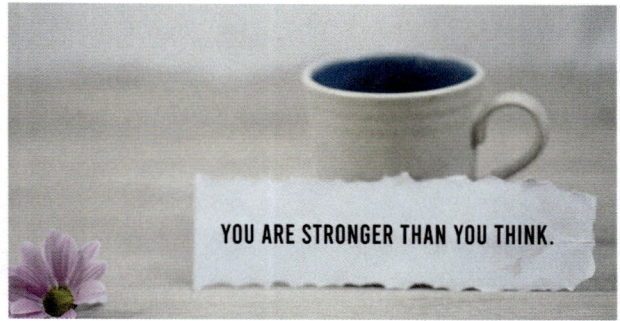

If, however, the words that you once heard, or are hearing now are feeding the thought that in some way you are not enough, **consider what might need to be eliminated, changed, or what support you can add.** Maybe, you have received positive feedback or felt that you were held to a higher standard than those around you. Does that place extra stress or pressure on you to try to be who or what someone else thinks you should be? Does it seem like there are expectations or assumptions of what you should do, who you should be, or what you should think, simply based on what you might be good at doing or might look like?

It is important to note that if the message is coming externally, from someone or something else, or a societal expectation, it is a bit of a different situation. If that is the case, pause. Decide if that is your issue or not. Ask yourself, are you expected to give more than enough, too much? If it is not your issue, if too much is being asked of you, it will never be fixed – it was not your issue to start with.

You have the power to choose to make a change for yourself.

Someone else changing is their responsibility.

Enough

Let us try and turn the focus back on ourselves and truly look at who and what we are, what we need, and what we like or want. Honestly, this might be one of the hardest things to do.

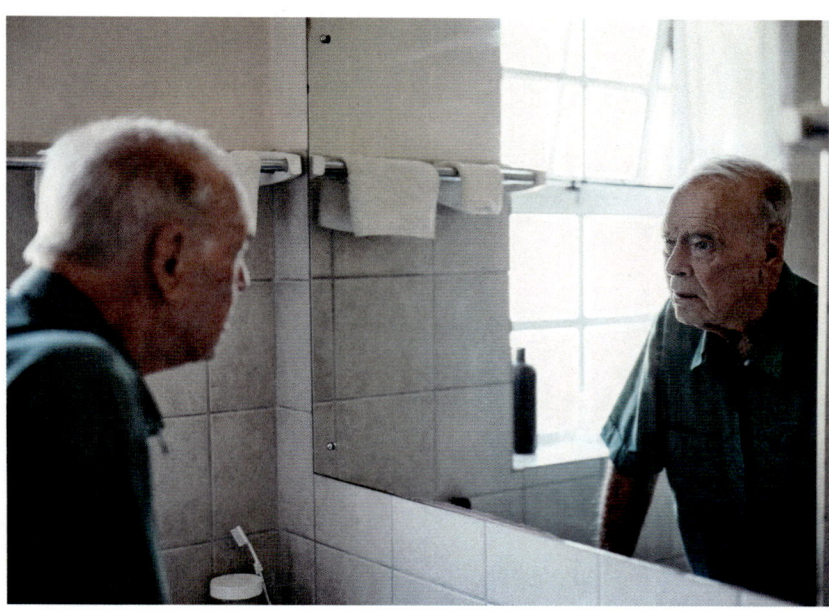

Maybe it is uncomfortable because when we look in the mirror, who is looking back? Are you seeing who you thought you would see? Are you seeing who you want to see?

Are you focusing on one specific problem area or are you noticing and taking into consideration the bigger picture of yourself? Your whole self?

Looking at ourselves, truly looking at ourselves, can be difficult. We know our strengths, our weaknesses, our vulnerabilities, but also our passions.

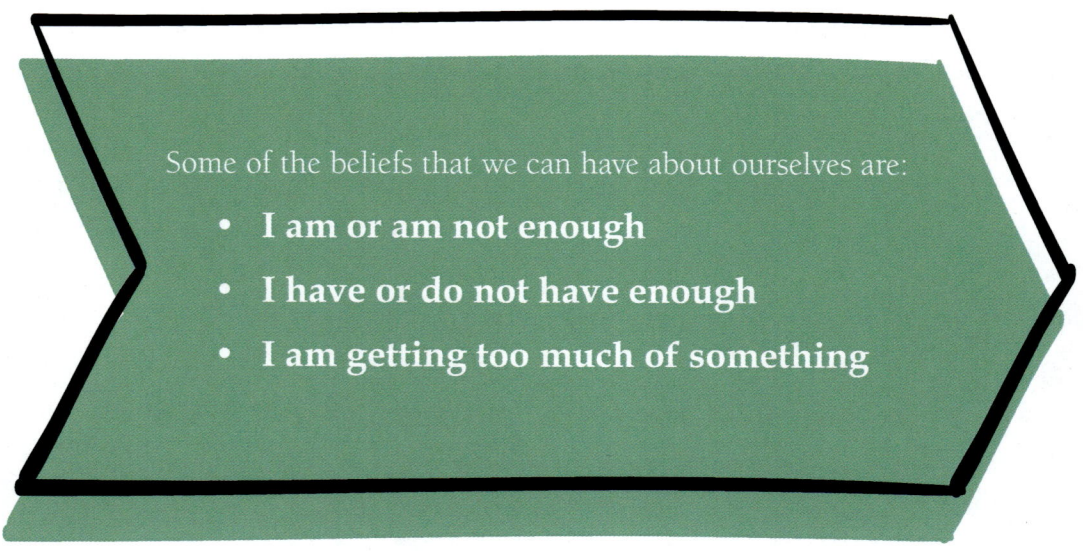

Some of the beliefs that we can have about ourselves are:
- I am or am not enough
- I have or do not have enough
- I am getting too much of something

Let us look a little deeper into what these beliefs might look like.

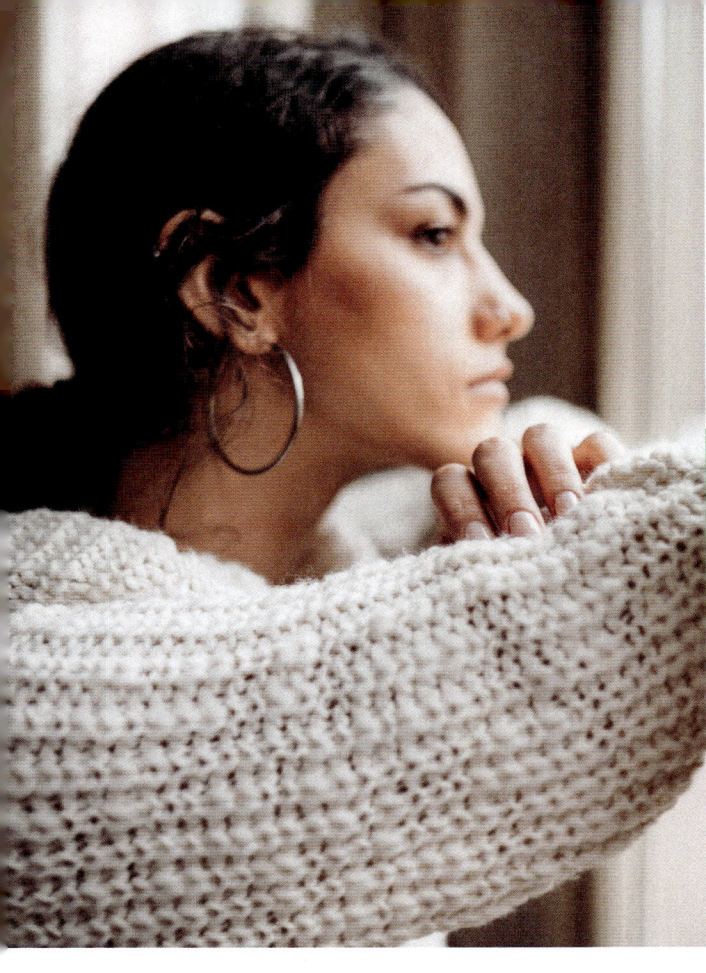

I am or am not enough

I am enough *–* I am giving what I need to give. I am confident and am balanced.

I am not enough *–* I am not giving or doing enough. I am not smart, rich, educated, happy, strong, brave, or attractive enough. I am not organized, creative, or caring enough.

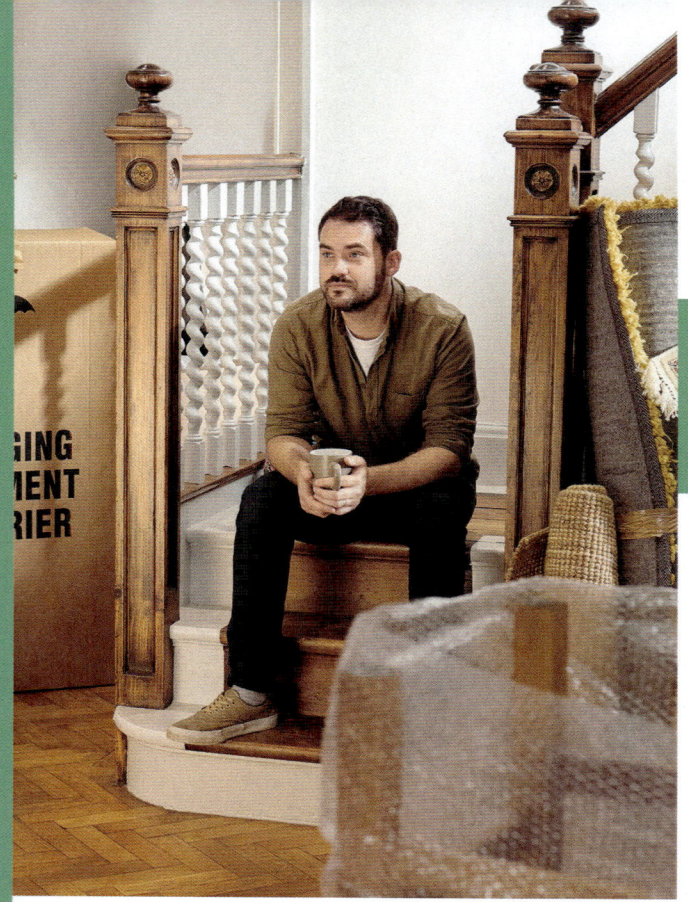

I have or do not have enough

I have enough – I am getting what I need and an acceptable amount of what I like and want. I am content and pleased with the things I own, the relationships I am in, and the support I have.

I do not have enough – I am not getting what I need. I do not have enough money, the right vehicle, the house I want, enough clothes, toys, or electronics. I do not have enough time for myself, for friends, or for work.

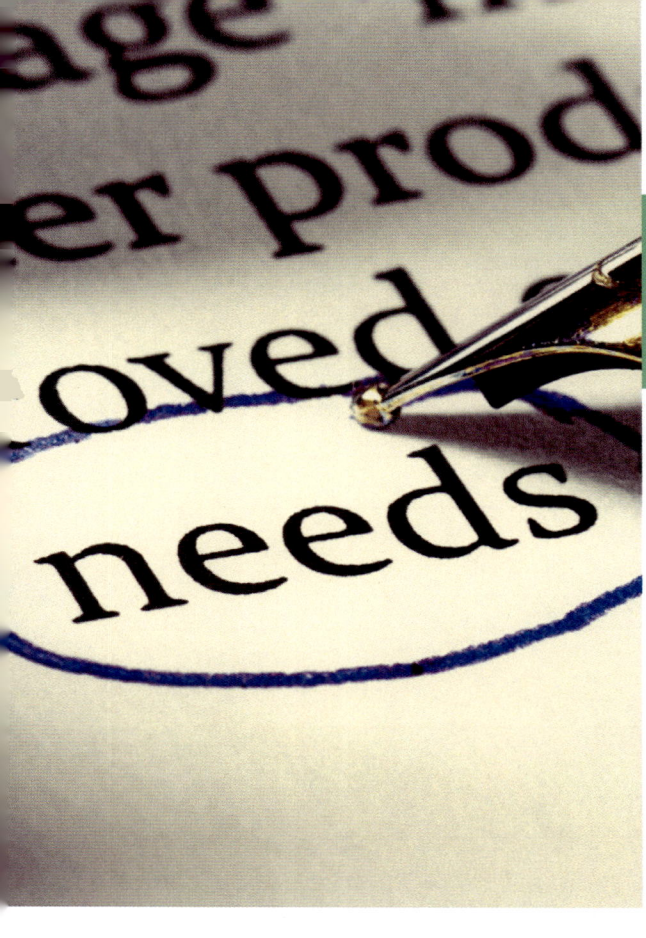

I am getting too much of something

I have HAD enough – I am getting too much of something. I do not like, want, or need what I am getting too much of. I am done, this is too much for me. There comes a point where too much is just too much. This can lead to frustration, discouragement, and sometimes even anger or resentment.

I have more than enough – I have a bountiful amount and I can share. **I have what I need and even what I want.** I am at a point where I can share with someone else and give them what I have.

You probably already have an opinion on how you are doing, what is it?

_____
_____
_____

What do you believe about yourself?

_____
_____
_____

Where is that belief coming from? Is it from someone else? If so, who?

_____
_____
_____

Can you identify a need that is not being met? If so, which one(s)?

_____
_____
_____

What is causing your need(s) to not be met?

_____
_____
_____

What is one thing you want to try differently to help meet your unmet need(s)?

_____
_____
_____

The idea of enough is all about the context around it. It is about whether something is balanced or not. To find balance and to stay balanced oftentimes requires us to shift our focus. **When things begin to seem unbalanced, what have you shifted your focus away from?**

_____
_____
_____
_____
_____

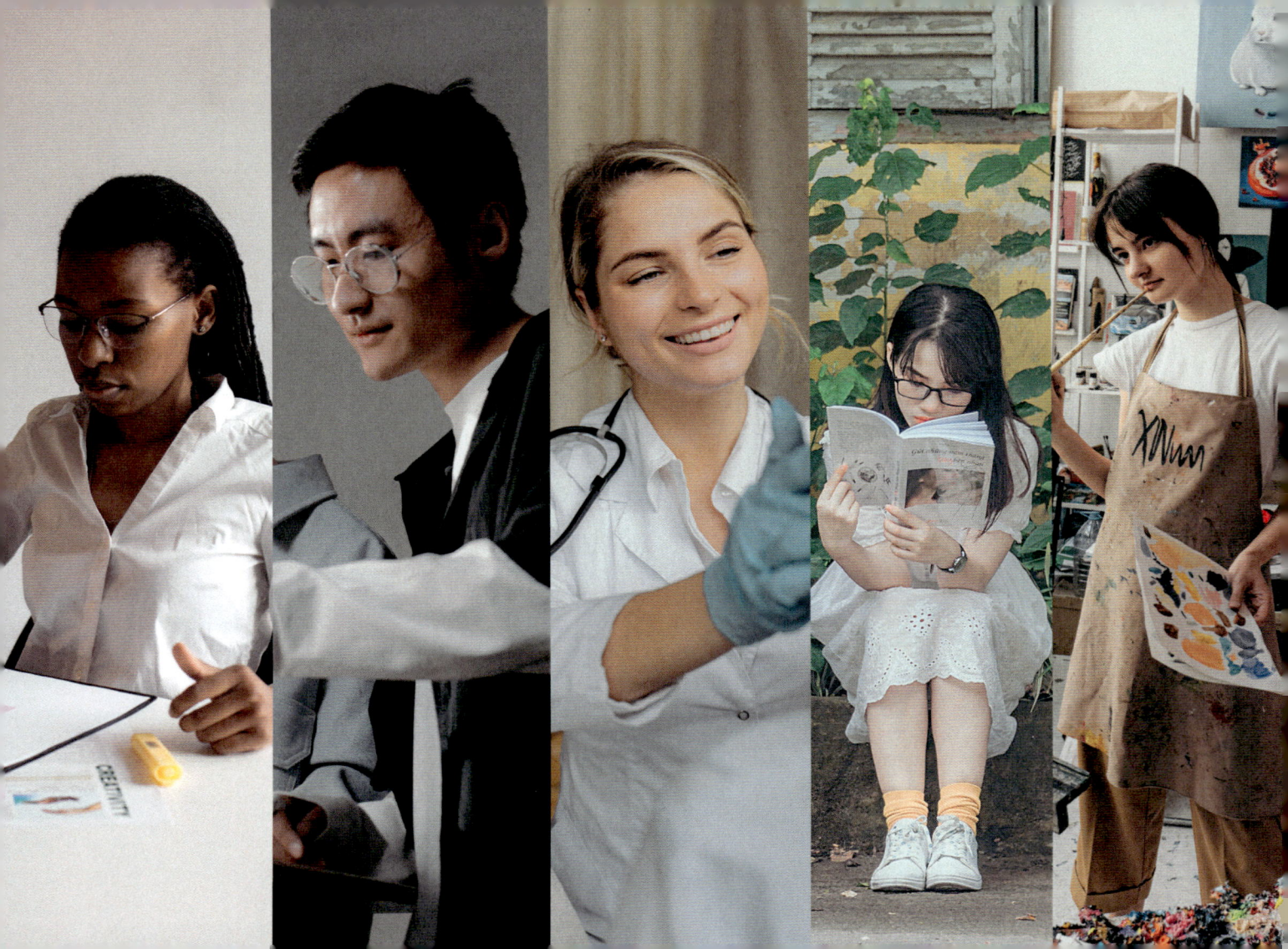

Personality Types

Over the past few pages, we took a deep dive into the beliefs we hold about ourselves, and where those beliefs originated. Were those pages an easy read? Did you thoughtfully answer each question or skip the whole section all together? Either way, it is okay, because **we all interpret and process this type of thing differently**, which is why we think there is value in talking about personality types.

Understanding and accepting that if we want to live well with ourselves and those around us, appreciating personality types and GEMS States is quite important. It is worth acknowledging that **if we are not working well with the people in our lives, we will have potential issues, and that is where the sense of being unbalanced comes into play.**

In *Relationships. Guidebook for Teepa Snow's Positive Approach to All Relations,* we uncover the value of understanding our own personality type so that we can strengthen relationships with the people in our lives. We also discover ways to connect with other people based on both of our GEMS States.

Figuring out what is enough, and what is the just right amount, all point back to finding balance. Here are a few thoughts on what each different personality type might need enough of to be balanced.

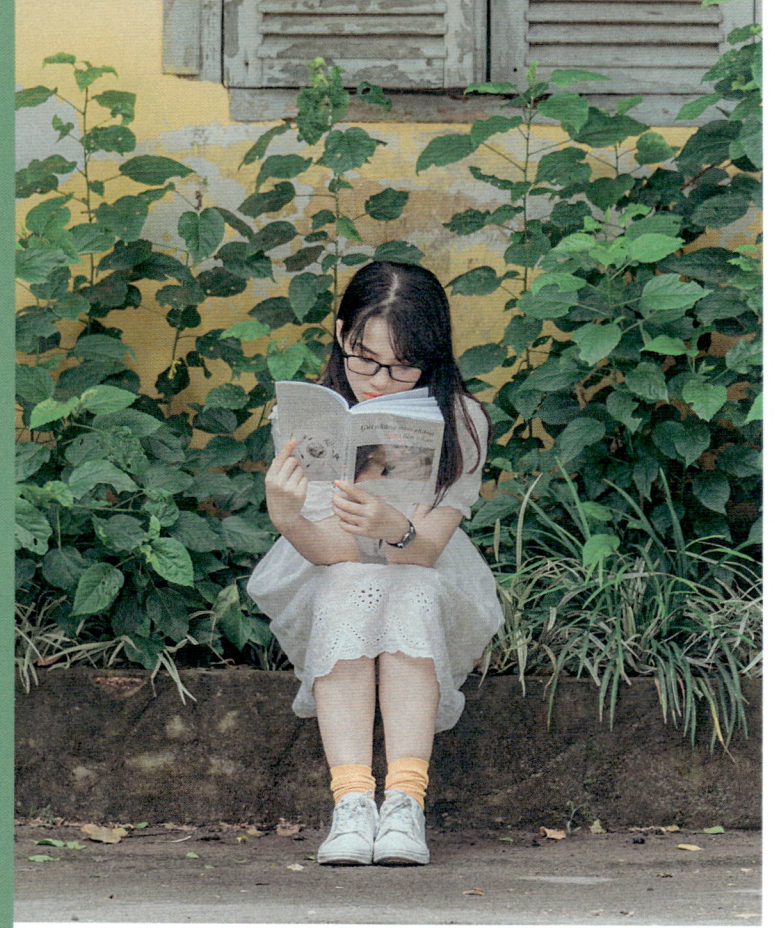

What an **introvert** tends to need enough of to be balanced:

- Alone time
- Privacy
- Plenty of time to think

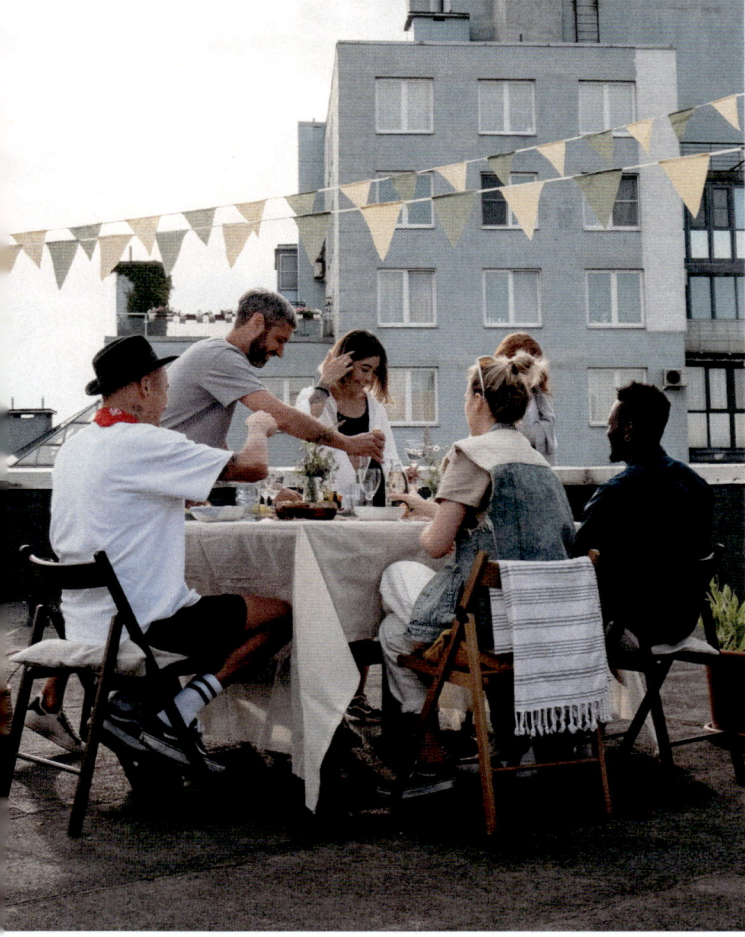

What an **extrovert** tends to need enough of to be balanced:

- Connection with a variety of people
- Time to talk
- Space to have others in their life around them

What about you? Are you an **introvert**, **extrovert**, or somewhere in the middle? What is enough for you? What does this mean for you as an individual or for the people you are trying to have a relationship with?

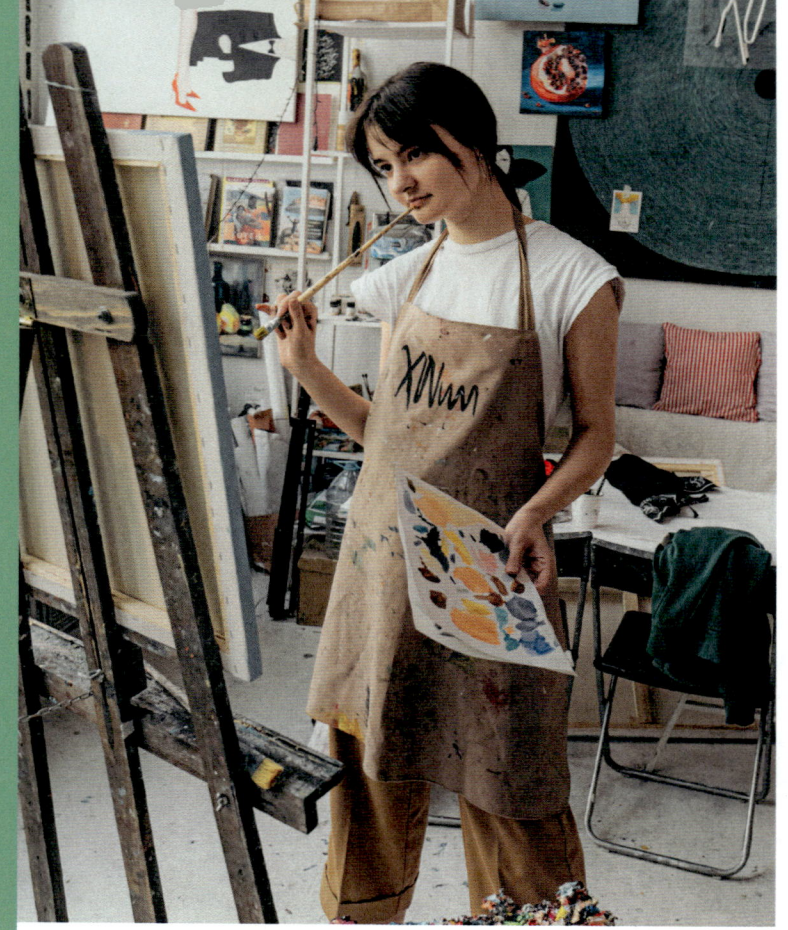

What a **why** person tends to need enough of to be balanced:

- Time and opportunity to try out options when doing something new or different
- Belief that there is value in what is being done
- The opportunity to recognize and appreciate the reason or meaning of what is being done prior to doing it

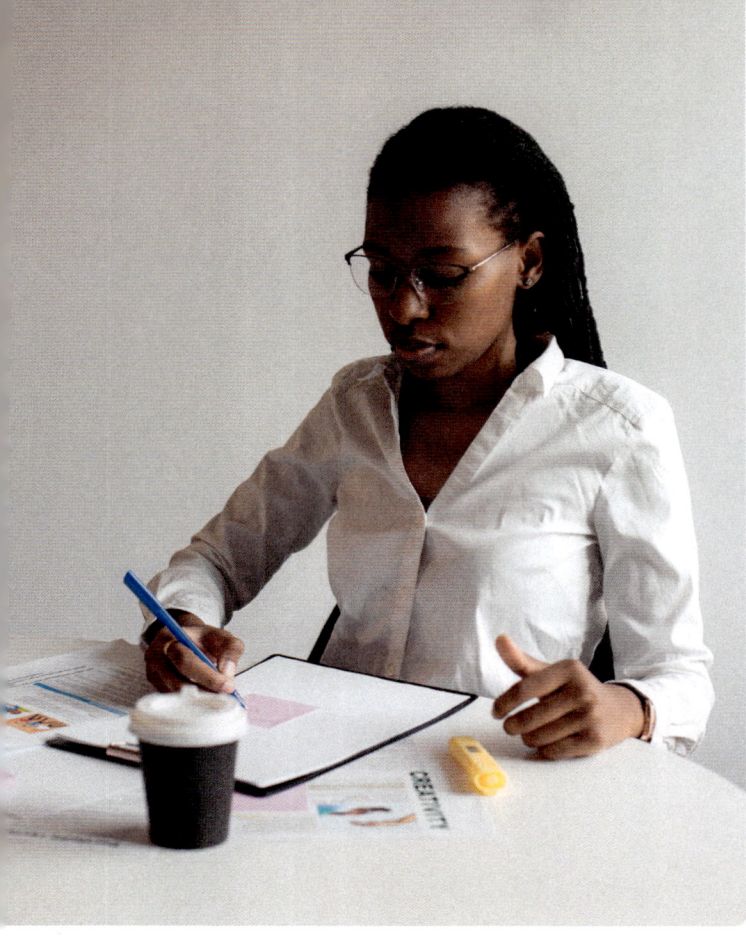

What a **how** person tends to need enough of to be balanced:

- Familiar tasks or activities
- Demonstrations or examples of something new
- Check lists or instructions

> **What about you?** Are you more **how, why,** or somewhere in the middle? What is enough for you? What does this mean for you as an individual or for the people you are trying to have a relationship with?

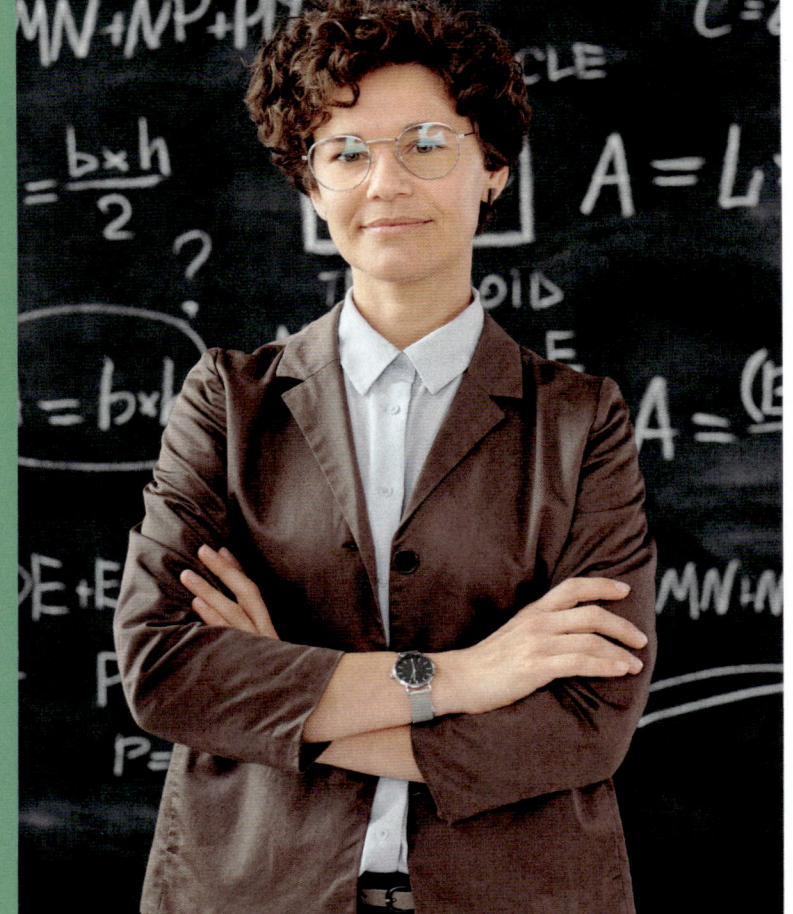

What a **head first** person tends to need enough of to be balanced:

- For something to make sense

- Some evidence or proof that something is fair and equal

- A sense that there is logic, reason, and facts being used before doing something or making a decision

When is Enough, Enough? *A Positive Approach to Finding Balance in a Caring Life*

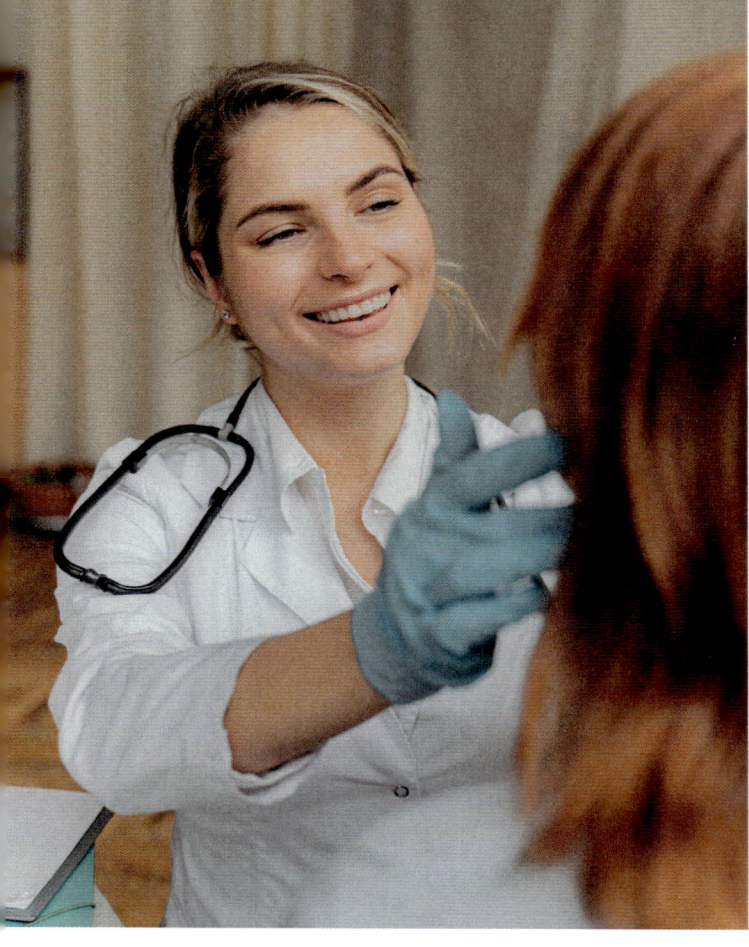

What a **heart first** person tends to need enough of to be balanced:

- A belief that people are feeling ok and are being taken care of
- An understanding of the cause of a problem
- An opportunity to create harmony between people

What about you? Are you more **head first, heart first,** or somewhere in the middle? What is enough for you? What does this mean for you as an individual or for the people you are trying to have a relationship with?

When is Enough, Enough? *A Positive Approach to Finding Balance in a Caring Life*

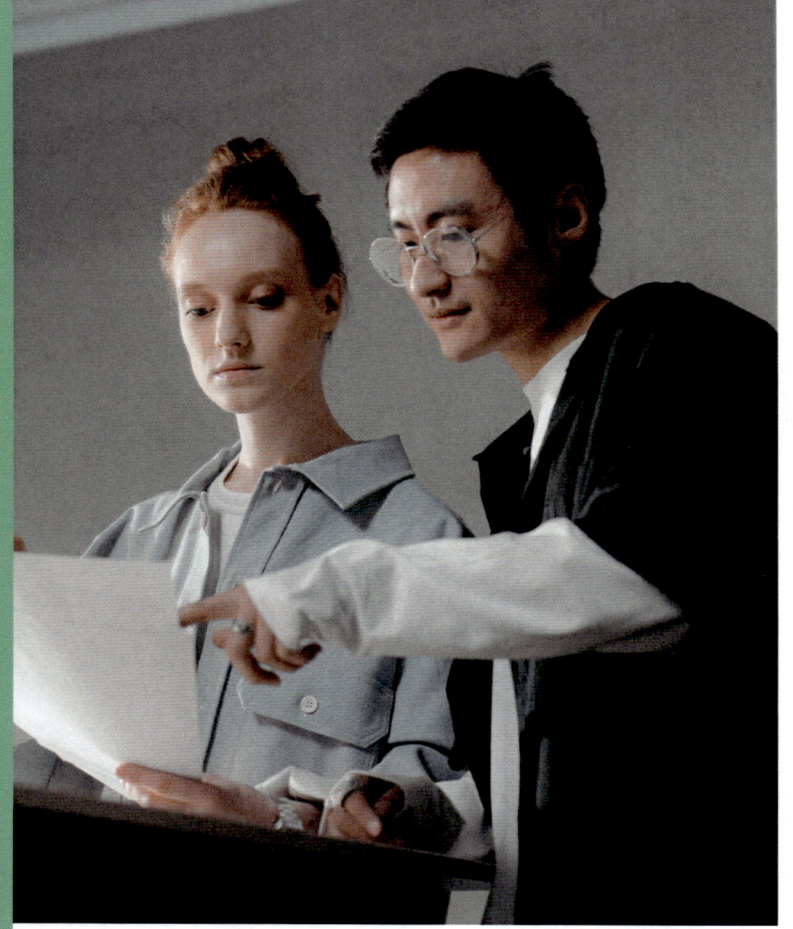

What a **plan ahead** person tends to need enough of to be balanced:

- Advanced notice and time to prepare
- A detailed plan that can be followed
- An understanding of what to expect and what is coming next

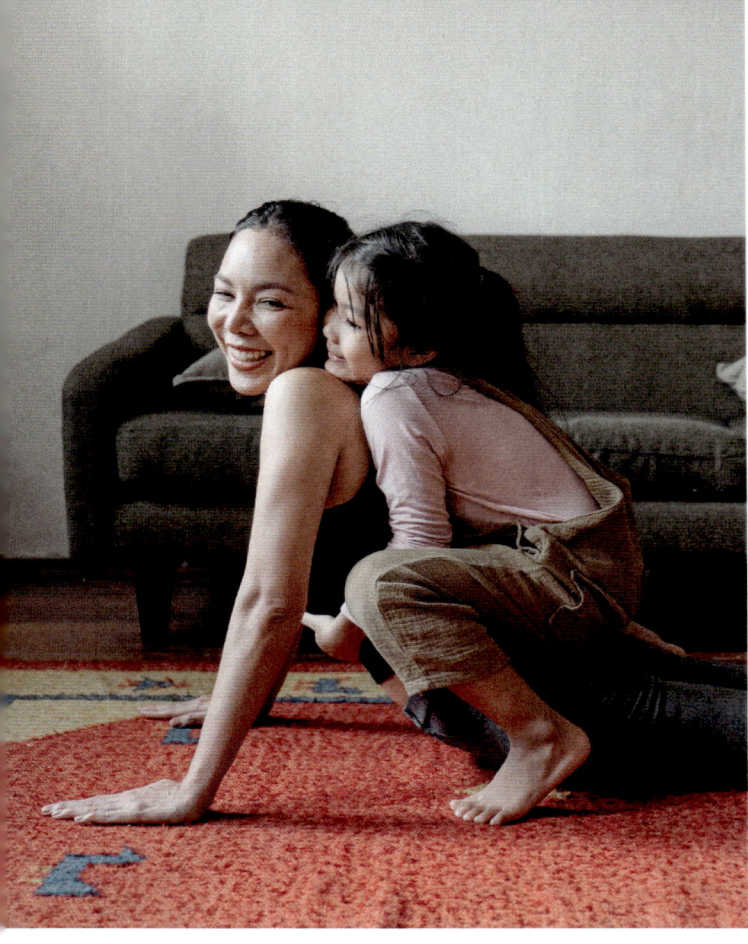

What a **live in the moment** person tends to need enough of to be balanced:

- Opportunities to identify what will be done or focused on at any moment. The ability to reprioritize based on what just happened

- Having flexibility in timelines and deadlines. Timelines are guidelines, not rules

- Flexibility with a schedule

> **What about you?** Are you more **plan ahead, live in the moment,** or somewhere in the middle? What is enough for you? What does this mean for you as an individual or for the people you are trying to have a relationship with?

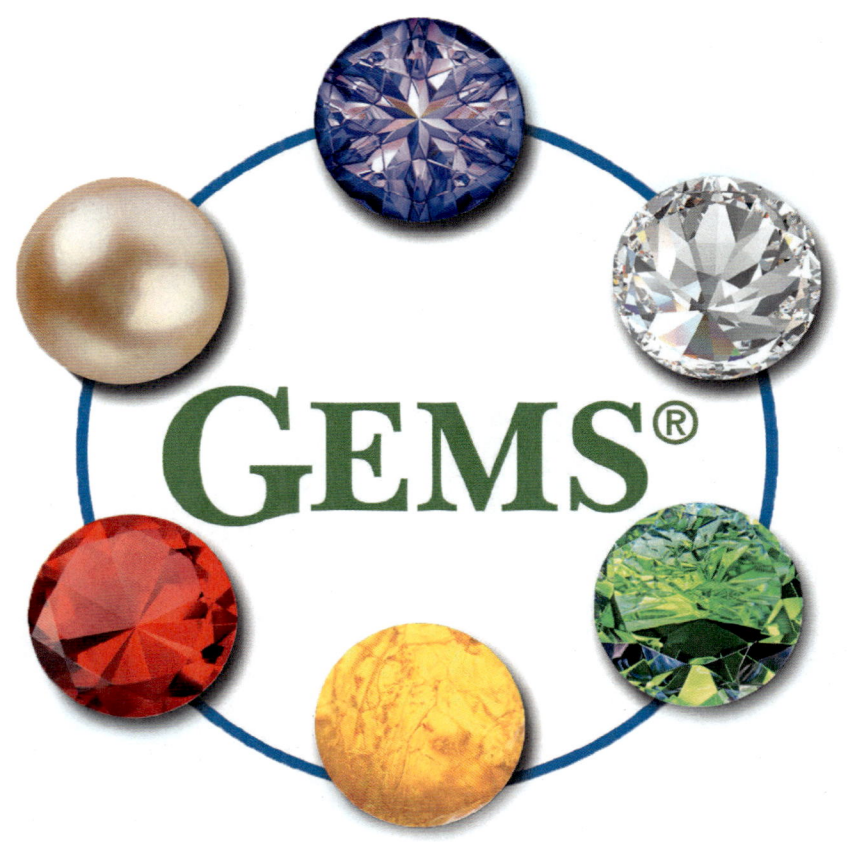

GEMS States

Now that we have looked at how different personality types might view being balanced, let us look at our different GEMS States. Our needs, physical, mental, emotional, and spiritual, especially when not met, can dramatically affect our GEMS State of mind. Furthermore, our GEMS State of mind can affect what we might do or say when something is out of balance. See? **It is all connected.**

In *Relationships. Guidebook for Teepa Snow's Positive Approach to All Relationships*, we explain that Teepa and her GEMS® State Model are best known when talking about brain change associated with dementia. There are specific chemical and physical changes that happen with dementia, but **all of us experience brain change day-to-day, hour-to-hour, minute-to-minute.** Teepa refers to them as States instead of stages because they are not fixed. We can, and do, move from one to another and back again, so it is truly a state of mind.

Each person, just like each gemstone, is precious, valuable, and unique.

Teepa Snow's GEMS State Model

 Sapphire – Flexible and adaptable. May find a way to adjust and become or stay balanced.

 Diamond – Clear and sharp. May need routine and familiar rituals of life to be balanced.

 Emerald – On-the-go and makes mistakes during transitions and/or initiating, sequencing, or completing a task. May need accurately offered support and guidance through transitions to be balanced.

 Amber – Looks for sensory experiences that are liked and avoids what is disliked. These sensory experiences guide actions, words, and interactions. Accuracy and judgement of what is enough becomes challenging as likes and wants are interpreted as needs. May need support and guidance to have needs met and to find balance.

Ruby – Calmed or excited by rhythm. Will need lots of help staying safe as needs are met and, together with a support person, balance may be found.

 Pearl – Resting or withdrawing into oneself. Will need lots of understanding, gentle support, and reassurance as, together with a support person, needs are met, and balance is sought after.

Each GEMS State will have unique patterns that help us figure out if they have not enough, too much, or just enough. **Enough is going to be where the person looks comfortable, satisfied, and is balanced.**

It is important to note that when it comes to the GEMS States, the idea of enough is a moving target. **Based on a person's GEMS State at a particular time, the perception of enough and balance may vary moment-to-moment.**

For a deeper look into the GEMS States, we encourage you to visit www.TeepaSnow.com.

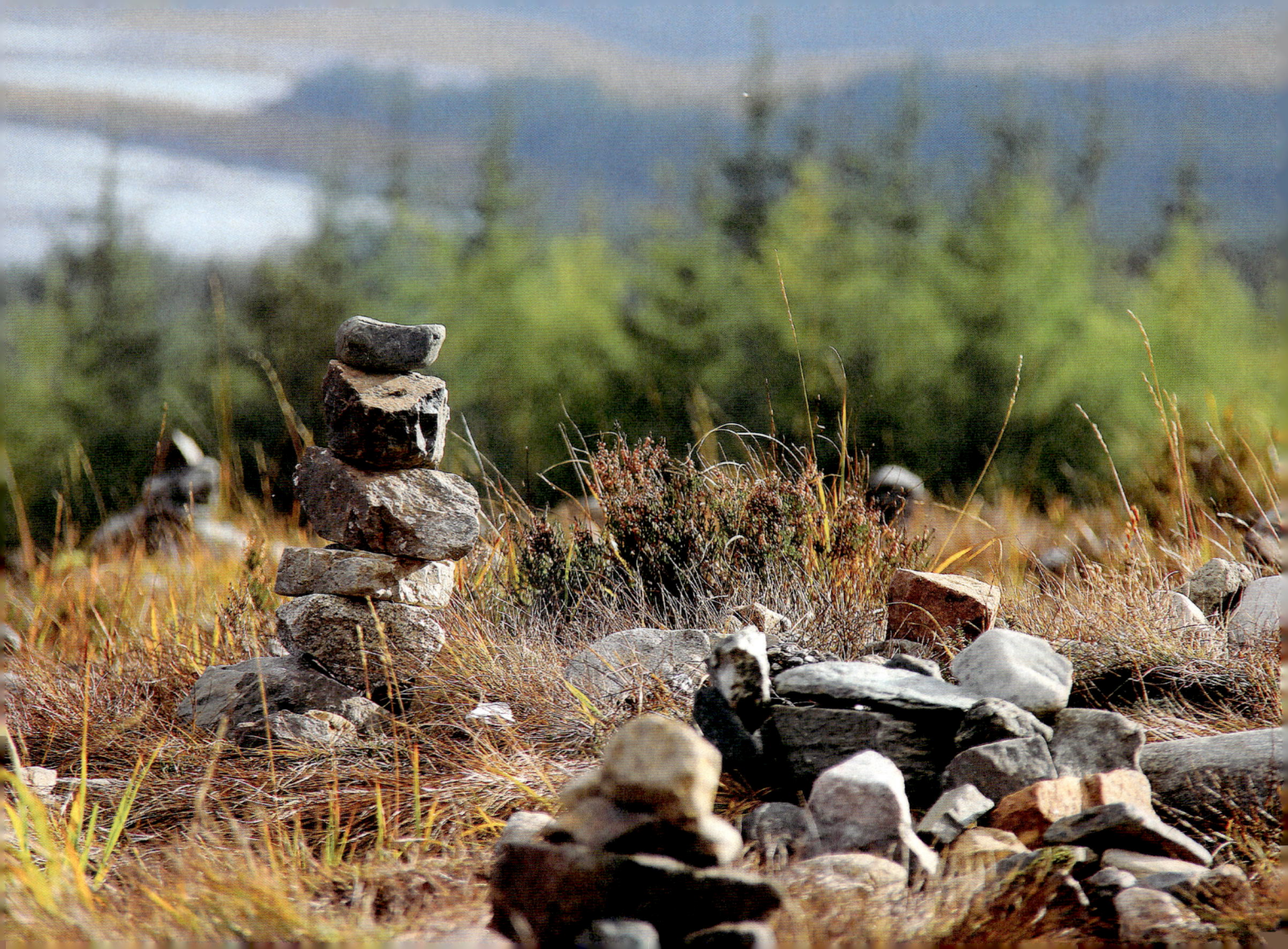

SECTION 3
Staying Balanced

How we help ourselves and the people around us live well, makes life worth living.

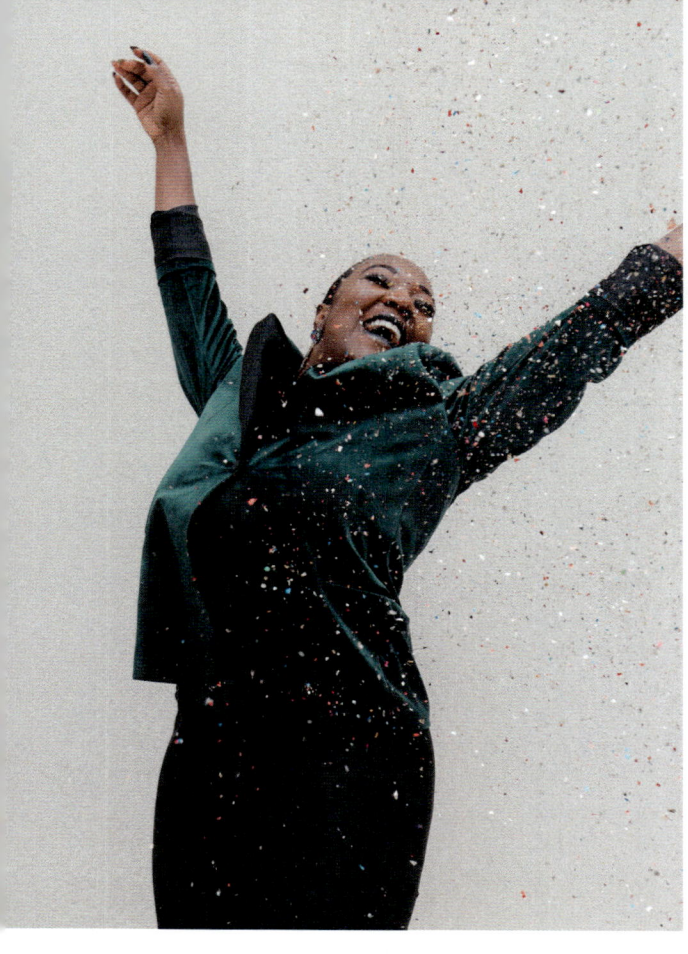

We have come a long way to get this far. Pat yourself on the back. Go ahead, be proud of the progress you have made. **You deserve it.**

So, now what? Where do we go from here? How do we continue to find balance and stay balanced in the middle of changes, relationships, or day-to-day events that are either expected or unexpected?

How do we realize and begin to appreciate that **enough is really where we should be?** To appreciate that joy comes in many ways and may only last for moments. Can we acknowledge moments of pain or discomfort while recognizing where our threshold is, being careful of what is tolerable before it becomes too much? While we would love for every moment to be joyful and absent of pain, we know that is not how life works. To be balanced, we need to try and hold on to those moments of joy and use them to help us work through the more difficult times.

The experiences of our lives help our brains, bodies, senses, and souls to mature. We can, over time, gain an appreciation for the value of having and not having enough. However, if we allow ourselves to limit our view of who we are, of who we can be, of others, and look at our world through too narrow a lens, we have the potential of developing patterns and habits that drive us further from a balanced life, and into one that is teetering on the edge.

Consider comparing resilience to rigid adherence and constant instability. Rubber bands and springs are designed to be stretched then relaxed so they can connect or contain different objects or items. If stretched to their limit, and kept there too long, fatigue sets in, and the flexibility feature fails. **The rubber band snaps and the spring fractures if the tension is not relieved or limited.** Just the same, **we are not meant to be static or stretched to our max repeatedly, only just enough to build resilience within our limits.**

Scan this code with your smartphone's camera
or visit **www.teepasnow.com/resources/enough-guide**
on your computer.

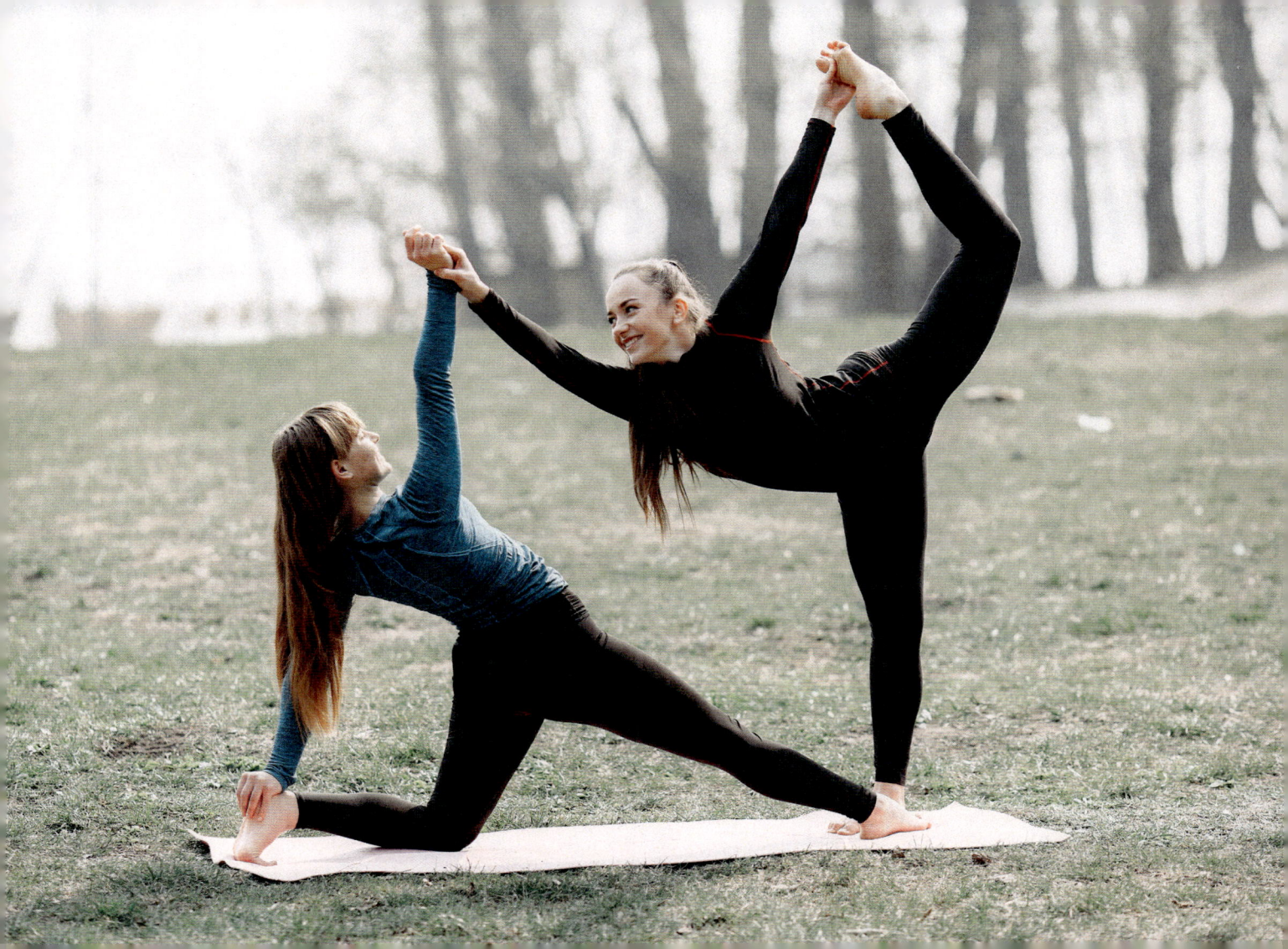

Consider these as steps we can seek to stay balanced:

- **Acknowledge** – Acknowledge when things are not going like you would like them to. Acknowledge when something does not seem right or when something is out of balance. Begin to recognize your own signals of being stretched to the max or reaching your limit. Do you notice it yourself, or is there someone who can help you pick up on the clues or cues? **Take time to let it be. It is what it is.**

- **Encourage** – Look around you and see who is on the journey with you. If it seems there is no one, consider who can come alongside you and offer you support. **Think of where, what, or who you turn to when you need help balancing, or perhaps a gentle reminder of your purpose, value, and worth.**

- Grow – Consider where you are putting your focus. **It is much easier to take a step forward when we are looking and focusing on what is in front of us.** You have a new level of awareness, and that alone is growth. Give yourself some wiggle room. Identify how to give someone else space enough to figure out and honor their own needs, while choosing to not take responsibility for the other person's needs being met. Realize that perhaps just reading this page is doing enough for right now. **If you choose to grow, you will grow.**

- Gratitude – Look around you. **What are you grateful or thankful for?** What can you offer up in thanks that was perhaps difficult or challenging? Consider this, many times it is by doing the hard thing or going through a tough situation that we learn more about ourselves and can build resilience. We certainly want to be grateful for the shining, special, and happy moments, but also consider being thankful for the stumbles, falls, trips, and mistakes. That is how we truly learn about ourselves, those around us, and what is possible. Be grateful for the opportunities to make mistakes that create a chance to develop a new skill or ability. If everything is always nice and smooth, we are not building resilience. **Look around and see what you have and appreciate that before looking at what else there could be.**

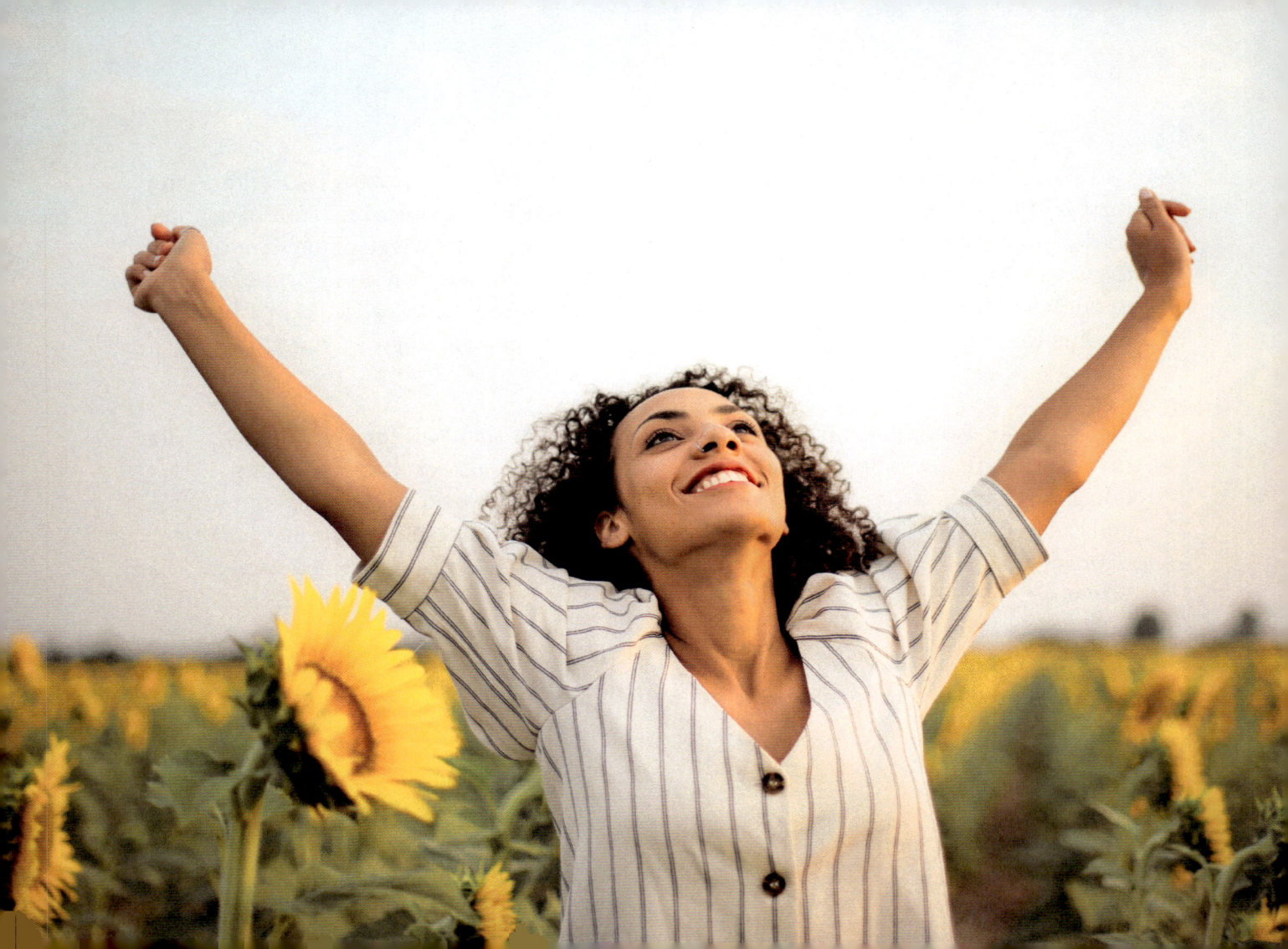

When we realize that we have a purpose, choose to find it, and live into it, there is freedom in that.

That is when we can share it and make a difference.

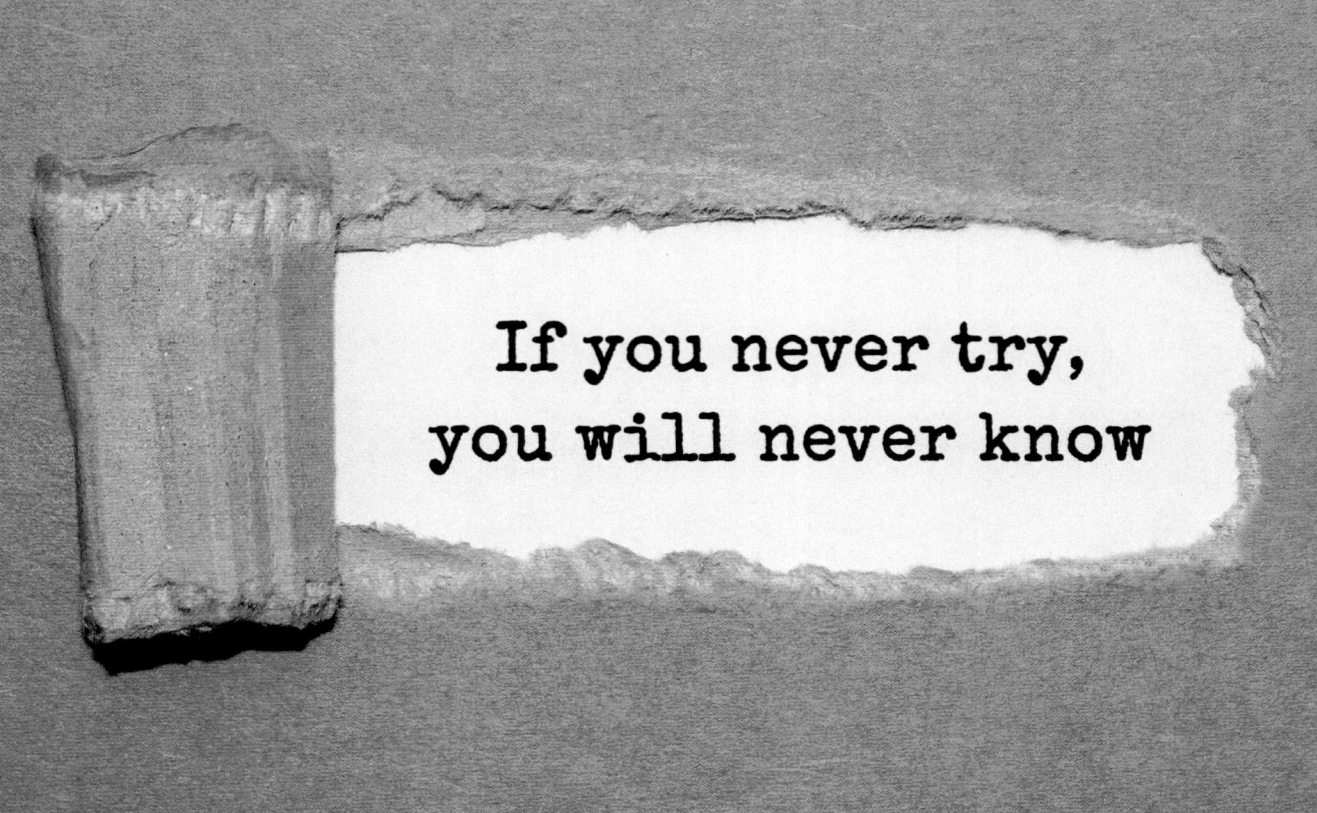

About the READY series

The second book in our five-part READY series. *When is Enough, Enough?* will help you find balance in all areas of your life by considering the five basic core human needs.

In order to improve or change a relationship, find balance, change a situation, do something different, or have a conversation, we must first be READY.

Relationships. *Positive Approach to All Relationships*

Enough. *When is Enough, Enough? Positive Approach to Finding Balance*

A *Coming Soon*

D *Coming Soon*

Y *Coming Soon*

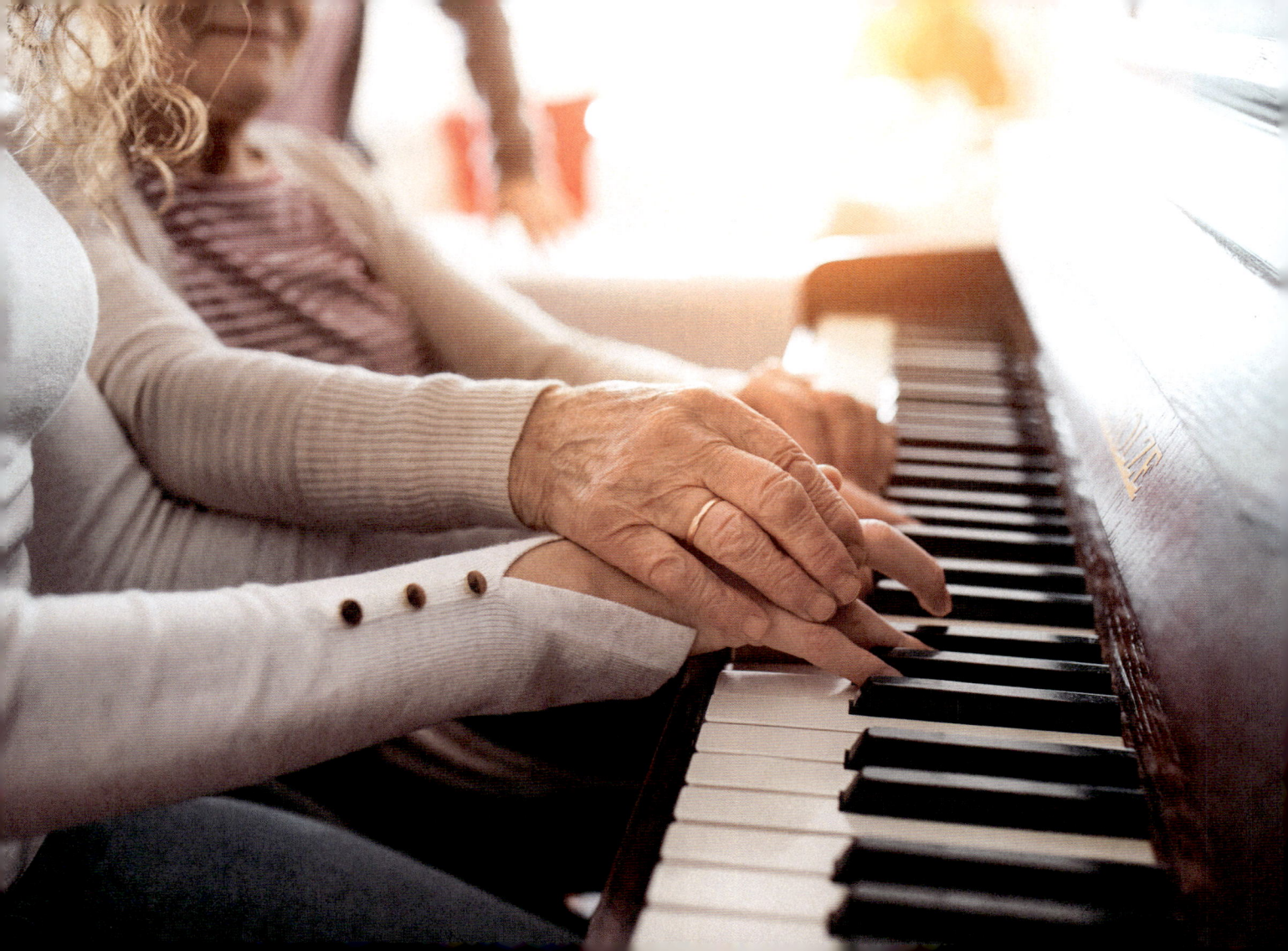

About Positive Approach to Care

Teepa's company, Positive Approach to Care (PAC), was founded in 2006 and is now collaborating to improve dementia care in over thirty countries worldwide. PAC provides online and in-person services, training, and products to professionals, family members, the lay public, and people living with brain change.

Please visit www.teepasnow.com for educational video clips, DVDs, books, information on individual certifications, online support groups, virtual and onsite trainings, or to subscribe to our free monthly newsletter.

Please also join us by liking and subscribing to:

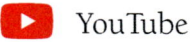 YouTube   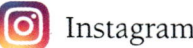 Instagram   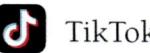 TikTok   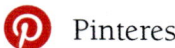 Pinterest

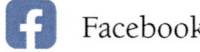 Facebook   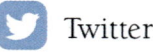 Twitter   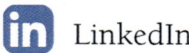 LinkedIn

General Resources

Thank you for reading this book and helping Teepa and her Positive Approach to Care team change the culture of dementia care, one mind at a time.

Teepa has created many products that can help you take the next steps in your awareness, knowledge, and skill in dementia care. Whether you are caring for someone living with dementia, living with dementia yourself, or part of a supportive community, there is something for you.

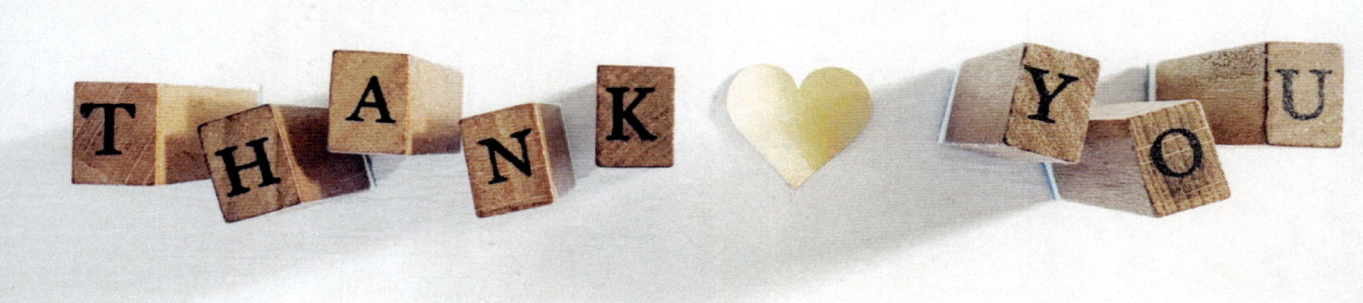

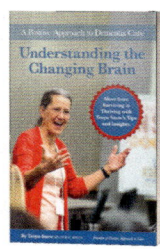 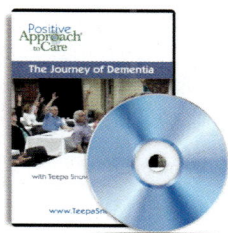  

Books. Teepa has written several books, all available on her website, www.teepasnow.com. Teepa's books focus on caregiving, relationships, music, dementia education for kids, and more.

Videos. Teepa has over 40 DVD titles, all of which are available in a DVD or online streaming format. Topics include bathing, end of life, types of dementia, selecting senior care, and many others.

Workshops. Whether you are looking to meet others who are in a similar situation, or learn and practice caregiving skills, we have something for you.

 There is someone to help you identify your next step. We are more than happy to help. You can reach us by phone at (877) 877-1671, or by email at info@teepasnow.com.

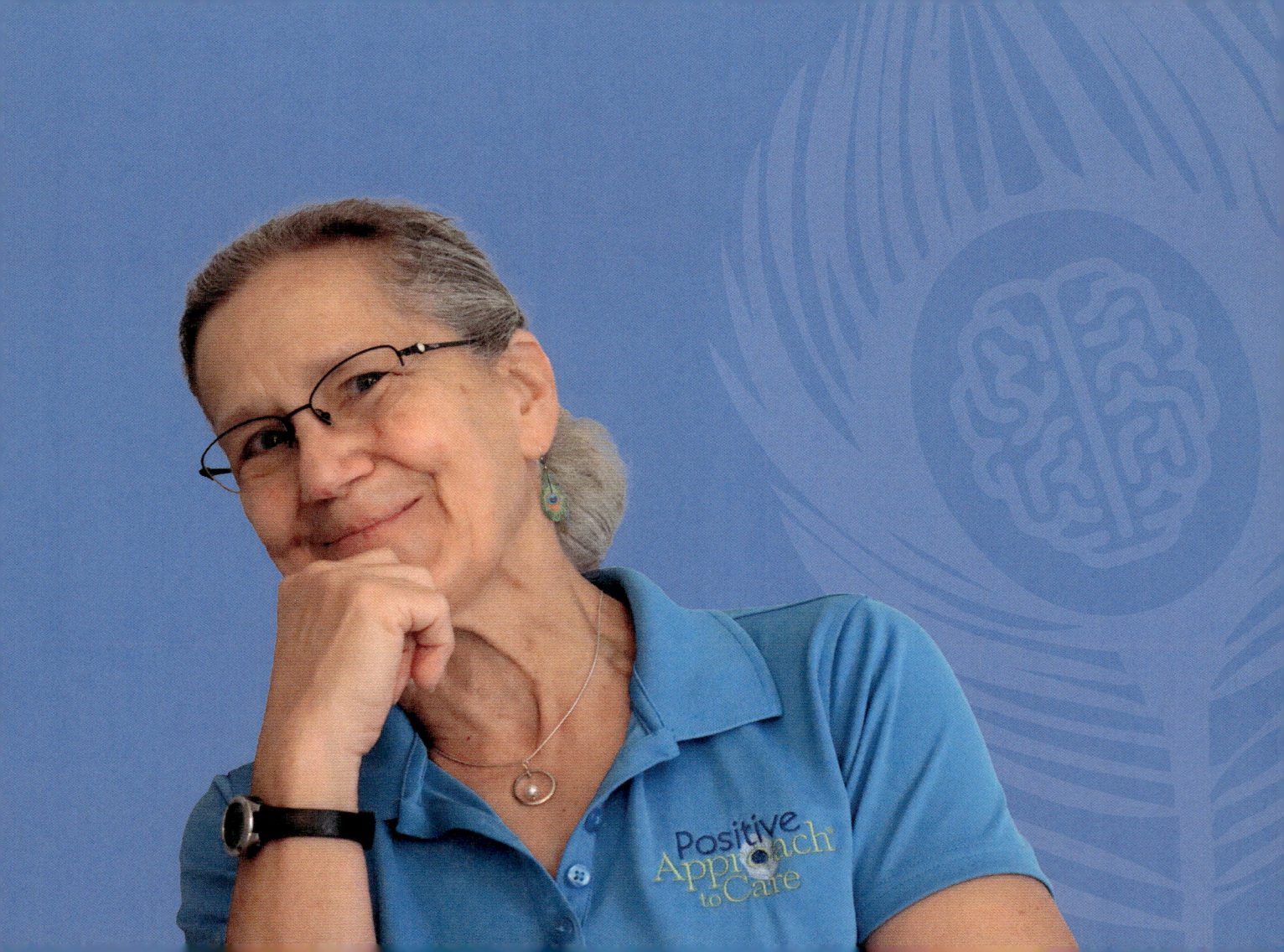

May your life be filled with just enough to satisfy, so you can be who and how you are meant to be on your journey.

Leepa L. Snow

Scan this code with your smartphone's camera
or visit **www.teepasnow.com/resources/enough-guide**
on your computer.

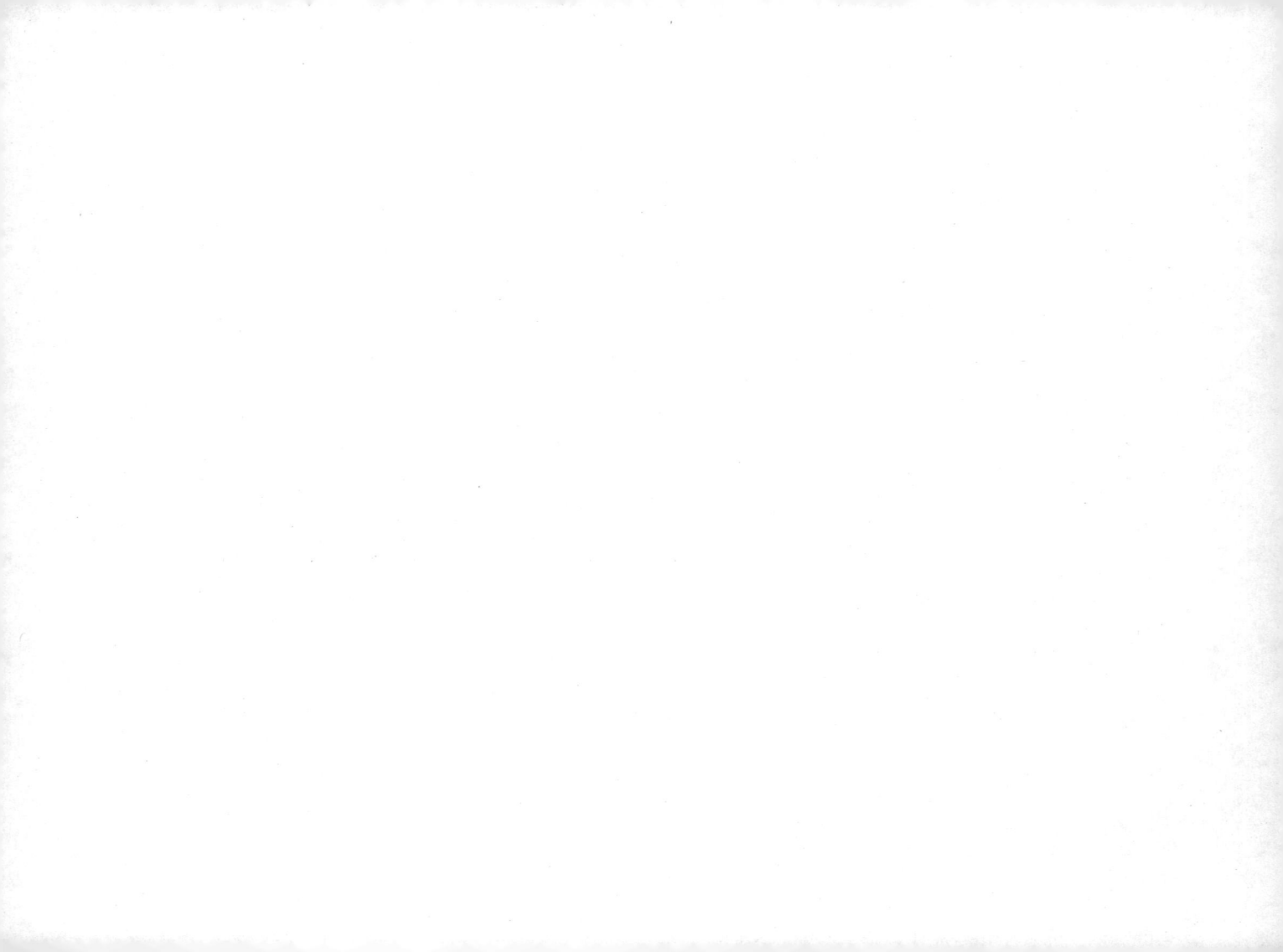

Made in the USA
Las Vegas, NV
11 December 2022

61896375R00057